Save Your Heart

Save Your Heart

ERNEST AEGERTER, M.D.

VAN NOSTRAND REINHOLD COMPANY
New York Cincinnati Toronto London Melbourne

Library of Congress Catalog Card Number 80-25288
ISBN 0-442-23112-1

Printed in the United States
Designed by Helene Berinsky
Line drawings by Radu Vero

Published by Van Nostrand Reinhold Company
135 West 50th Street
New York, NY 10020

Van Nostrand Reinhold Limited
1410 Birchmount Road
Scarborough, Ontario MlP 2E7, Canada

Van Nostrand Reinhold Australia Pty. Ltd.
17 Queen Street
Mitcham, Victoria 3132, Australia

Van Nostrand Reinhold Company Limited
Molly Millars Lane
Wokingham, Berkshire, England

16 15 14 13 12 11 10 9 8 7 6 5 4 3 2 1

Library of Congress Cataloging in Publication Data
Aegerter, Ernest Emil, date
How to save your heart.

Includes index.
1. Atherosclerosis—Nutritional aspects.
2. Atherosclerosis—Diet therapy. 3. Heart—Diseases —Prevention. I. Title. [DNLM: 1. Diet, Reducing exertion—Popular works. 2. Arteriosclerosis—Prevention and control—Popular works. 3. Diet, Atherogenic—Popular works. WG 550 A247h]
RC692.A33 616.1′3605 80–25288
ISBN 0-442-23112-1

To Florence

Contents

Put a knife to thy throat if thou be a man given to appetite.

—PROVERBS

Introduction

Any good bookstore can boast at least a hundred different cookbooks. There are several from nearly every nationality of the world and just about every geographic and political division of the United States. There are cookbooks for various eras, climates, altitudes, and incomes. There are even cookbooks for different marital states and sexual preferences. I found in my favorite bookstore a host of books concerned with low-calorie menus and at least a few on how to cook with a limited amount of fat. What I did not find was a comprehensive and practical book on the types and preparation of foods low in both calories and animal fat.

In the course of this book, you will read that you can reduce your weight by limiting your intake of calories, but you will not thereby greatly reduce your chances of dying of one of the most common causes of death—myocardial infarction (heart attack), cerebrovascular accident (stroke), or hypertension (high blood pressure)—which are caused by or associated with the condition known as atherosclerosis. If, on the other hand, you adhere to a diet devoid of animal fat, you may escape atherosclerosis but suffer from obesity and discover that overweight is also associated with these same fatal diseases. This book attempts to remedy the curious and widespread lack of knowledge of the most important things people should be doing to enjoy a long and healthful life: avoiding atherosclerosis and obesity. Occasionally a fat person enjoys his obesity, but the obese, too, hope to live their anticipated three score and ten. Why, then, have so many people remained uninformed about the perils of atherosclerosis?

As a physician who has spent many years teaching the basic medical sciences, I became aware long ago that although most people know very little about their anatomy and how it functions, most of them have a genuine desire to learn. I have not written at length about the chemistry and physiology of the human body; I have left that to those medical professionals who make it their business. Nonetheless, I hold that the average person should know as much about how his body works as he does about how his automobile works. Particularly, he should know the basic facts about the fuel and maintenance that are necessary to promote a long and healthy life and about the pitfalls that are almost sure to curtail it.

A regimen of proper diet and exercise requires little more than motivation and a modicum of self-discipline. It has always been my belief that people find discipline a lot easier when they understand the reasons for it and especially when they know how they can benefit from it. That is why this book is not simply a collection of menus and recipes. This is not a cookbook. You will find some recipes that are meant to illustrate the manner in which you may enjoy a truly healthful diet, but essentially this is an account of how your tissues utilize the food you supply them, what types of foods are good for you, and which foods you should make every effort to avoid. Moreover, I have tried to explain why animal fats are deleterious and to suggest some substitutes that make the elimination of fats from the diet less onerous.

Nor is this a "doctor's book" in which an alphabetical listing of symptoms is provided for reference when you are ailing. Such books are dangerous and rarely used in this country because professional help is so widely available, if expensive.

It is my belief that most people want to know the basic facts about atherosclerosis and how it causes or is related to conditions that cause the death of about six out of every ten of us. Most people feel that they have a right to know as much as physicians do about how to avoid this condition in order to increase longevity. I believe that most people will appreciate the threat and be better prepared to deal with it if they understand how it is brought about. I have tried to present this material in a way that will not seem tedious to anyone who does not have a detailed knowledge of anatomy and physiology. I can assure you that the knowledge you glean from these pages may be the most rewarding of any you have attained.

It is my sincere belief, based on years of study and experience, that the incidence of atherosclerosis can be decreased and its severity reduced by observing the type of diet recommended in this book. It is my belief too that the aging process may be slowed, and that the person nourishing his tissues on a low-fat diet has a better chance of enjoying a longer and more active life. If this seems a worthwhile objective, then the effort put forth to understand the material that the medical sciences have provided over the past two decades is little enough. And if the discipline required to learn to enjoy the food that will bring you health and freedom from atherosclerosis and premature aging at first seems odious, promise of its eventual rewards will keep you close to the line of sane diet behavior.

There are two acknowledgments that should be made in grateful appreciation for the help received writing this book; to John Andrews Duross, *chef extraordinaire*, who did much of the menu and recipe research, and to Barbara Kelman-Burgower, the most intelligent and considerate editor with whom I have ever worked.

1

Join the Revolution

Six out of ten of us will die of a disease that probably can be prevented by eating properly. The disease I speak of is atherosclerosis, by far the most significant of a number of diseases related to the quantity and quality of the food we consume. Obesity, high blood pressure, and stroke are among the other important diet-related diseases.

If we are to reverse the trend, we must revolutionize our eating habits. Let us change the watchword of this revolution from "we live to eat" to "we eat to live!"

It is perhaps ironic that the changes we must make in our habits of food consumption are necessitated by positive factors of modern life, among them the longevity achieved over the past century. When people could expect to die at the age of forty-five of infections such as pneumonia, peritonitis, tuberculosis, typhoid fever, diphtheria, and syphilis, few had the time to develop lethal atherosclerosis. Now, with increasing numbers of people reaching seventy-two and older, there is plenty of time and ample opportunity.

When we take a long look at our potential life span we should realize that we must change our dietary habits to realize our possibilities. Today all of us should seriously consider joining this revolution before it is too late.

Atherosclerosis, a type of arteriosclerosis or "hardening of the arteries," is the cause of, or a major factor in, coronary heart disease, stroke, gangrene of the extremities, kidney failure, hypertension, and senile dementia. Most of us will have a degree of one or even most of these ailments, and more than half of us will die as a result. Obesity is another killer because it makes us susceptible to hypertension. It is a sneaky menace that sets the trap for other, more scrutable predators. What and how much you eat certainly determines your weight. Your weight and the kind of food that maintains it are factors in the development of a number of diseases, including atherosclerosis.

For many years and for many people, a typical breakfast has consisted of fruit juice, cereal, one or another kind of pork (bacon, sausage, or ham), eggs, and toast with marmalade. Today, more sensible people have a cup of coffee (often black) on rising and another when they reach their place of work. Dinners have undergone changes almost as radical. When I was quite young I expected a bowl of soup at dinner time, a meat dish and two vegetables, often a salad, and always a dessert. It was served promptly at six o'clock. Now most of my thinner, more active friends partake of an ample serving of a meat dish, a vegetable, and often a salad at about eight o'clock. Today food is more interesting and imaginative; it is more varied and served in smaller portions. We must see to it, however, that it is also less fattening and less atherogenic (tending to cause atherosclerosis).

Achieving these changes requires a culinary revolution. Our grandparents would probably protest, but science, medicine, and unbiased intelligence are now shouting loud and clear, and in unison at last: if you cling to your breakfast eggs, your chocolate sundae at lunch, and a roast with pan gravy for dinner, you had better straighten up and fly right.

Many people are ignorant of basic nutritional facts; others are the victims of counselors who are more interested in their own compensation than in the welfare of their clients or customers. But knowledge of the facts is often not enough. I know a gentleman who has had a serious bout with coronary heart disease. He did survive the attack, but was told that he had to reduce sharply his fat intake. Egg yolk may not be the most important contribution to atherosclerosis (although we think it probably is, we still lack incontrovertible proof), but as far as my friend knows, it is. Nonetheless, he continues to enjoy his two eggs for breakfast every morning—without his physician's knowledge. Yes, we may know the facts, but how many of us will conform to their dictates?

What would you do if you knew you had less than a 50 percent chance of avoiding being attacked and gobbled up by an alligator? It is reasonable to assume that you would avoid zoos and never go for a boat ride in the Everglades. In the following pages I shall try to convince you that this is more than a psychedelic nightmare, and that unless you heed the portents I am about to proclaim you had better prepare for the inevitable.

The name of your alligator is arteriosclerosis, the thickening and deterioration of your arterial system that leads to a number of diseases, the aggregate of which kills about twice as many people as die of cancer, cirrhosis, and automobile accidents combined. Almost everyone past middle age has some degree of atherosclerosis, the most common type of arteriosclerosis, and more than 50 percent of us will die of one or more of its complications. It is probably safe to say that the reason more people are not killed by alligators is that most of us are a bit reluctant to consort with the beasts. With atherosclerosis it is quite different; until recently most of us have had little choice. Now I think we have. That is what this book is about; a guide to how to use your good common sense and reasonable discipline to prolong your life.

Man eats too much!

He does so because he has circumvented one of nature's most fundamental regulations. He has managed to get away with breaking this law, but he has suffered from its backlash.

From the very beginning of time, the animal populations of the earth have been limited by their food supply. When you plant a rose garden you can expect to have an abundant crop of Japanese beetles. It has always been so. We have reduced the acreage of the grazing areas of our great central plateau and the herds of buffalo have disappeared. These are man-made confirmations of one of nature's most zealously enforced laws.

Almost all wildlife breeds to the supportive capacity of its supply of nourishment. Nature is a callous manager but an accurate bookkeeper. A few thousand lives, whether they be whooping cranes or *Homo sapiens*, do not much matter, but they are recorded on nature's abacus in order to keep all natural phenomena in order. When a year of plenty produces a bounty of foliage, berries, seeds, and nuts, the number of small wildlife, birds, and rodents increases. The opposite is true in a lean year. In short, because their numbers are regulated by their food supply, almost all animals in the wild state are constantly hungry and never fat. Only man and his parasitic population of lower forms—his domesticated livestock and pampered pets—have an opportunity to become obese. Nature has had her revenge. Obesity is a disease.

Man eats the wrong kind of food!

Before man came down from the trees, he lived largely on leaves, berries, and nuts. Over several million years, his cells developed a set of enzymes that could metabolize (break down and burn) plant carbohydrates (sugars and starches), plant proteins, and a few unsaturated fats (largely from seeds and nuts). Our ancestors lived in an arboreal environment and utilized its products; they were herbivorous (vegetarians). If you've tried such diets you know that they may become boring, so our tree-dwelling forebears probably achieved variety by mixing in an insect here, a tree toad there, and possibly the gourmets among them tried a bird or two for sheer exoticism. These additions were mostly protein and fat. The enzymatic equipment of these early experimenters could handle the protein admirably, but they must have had difficulty with the fats—particularly the saturated ones, because the cellular enzymes could not break them down completely for burning. Put to the task, these enzymes combined lipids (fats) with phosphates (protein constituents) to form a variety of molecules, some of greater density than others. The metabolic economy of the upright apes survived, but not efficiently. The low-density molecules tended to clog the metabolic pathways, to collect in unwanted rubbish heaps (atherosclerotic plaques) in the arteries. This debris caused obstruction of the blood supply to vital tissues. A host of complications ensued, and nature had her revenge.

Atherosclerosis is not wholly understood, but enough facts

have emerged to make it mandatory for everyone to do what he can to prevent it. I am convinced that matters of self-discipline are much easier to discharge when one has a sound reason for doing so. Reason is the daughter of knowledge. If we know the nature and function of our arterial system, we are better prepared to deal with its weaknesses—and ours in relation to it.

When faced with the possibility of a catastrophe at the hands (or jaws) of an alligator, the prudent avoid confrontation with the monster. The intelligent person should treat atherosclerosis with the same caution. I fully believe that this book will be helpful for those who consider thoughtfully the message contained herein.

2

Your Heart and Its Vessels

At the dawn of evolution, animals were all one-celled and lived in the sea. The getting and spending of life's necessities were simple matters. The cells took what they wanted from their environment, used what they needed, and cast the wastes back into the water around them. That system worked very well in a unicellular world. But nature has never been satisfied to leave things as they are. These unicellular animals began to specialize. One developed a set of chemicals called enzymes which allowed it to metabolize foods that others could not. Another learned to project footlike extensions of its body that enabled it to creep about on the slimy floor of its homeland, and a third specialized in extending these protrusions to ensnare smaller animals that could be used as food. These last were the original hunters.

"Now if I put these cells together," thought nature, "I'll have a single animal that is better than any of the three." And so she did.

It worked so well that she tried ever larger aggregates of cells, and then the trouble began. No longer had all the cells free surfaces exposed to their environment; instead, most were surrounded by contiguous cells. The only food and oxygen available to these interior cells was that discarded by neighboring cells. In order for larger animals to evolve, a transport system for food and oxygen had to be devised. There was already a model in the plant kingdom.

The evolution of plant life was evidently well advanced before the development of multicellular animals. As soon as chlorophyll came into being, photosynthesis (the conversion of solar to biologic energy) and the development of multiple-unit complexes of plant cells became possible. A current of fluid passes continuously through all living plants by means of capillary action. Water is taken from the soil through the plant's hair roots, ascends through microscopic channels between the plant cells in the stem, and is dissipated into the atmosphere through the leaves, whose high ratio of surface to mass promotes evaporation. This current of water carries essential nutrients and minerals extracted from the soil, and it allows the cells that it bathes to select what they need, just as their progenitors selected their needs from sea water.

The multicellular animal has the same problem as the multicellular plant, but more severe; the animal has no constant and inexhaustable fluid supply because it is motile, and it gains little benefit from evaporation because, lacking leaves, it has a very low surface to mass ratio. The transport system could be a fluid, but that fluid would have to be recycled so it could be used over and over again. Such a system requires a pump. The heart and its complex network of vessels were devised to supply the cells of the motile animal with food and oxygen.

The heart is the only organ in the body that constantly manifests its function; you are always aware of its existence. Perhaps because of this, the heart has come in for a lot of imaginative speculation. Cannibals have eaten it, claiming that it gave them vigor; the Aztecs cut it out of captive youths while still alive in a grisly sacrifice. Warriors of the middle ages believed the heart to be a fountain of courage, and Victorians considered it the symbol of love. They stylized the emblem into a valentine which, come to think of it, is a pretty macabre idea. Actually, the heart is only a piece of muscle fashioned into a four-chambered bulb with valves so arranged that when the heart contracts, fluids are pumped in two separate and distinct circuits, the systemic and pulmonary circulations.

Each circuit has an arterial and a venous system. The arter-

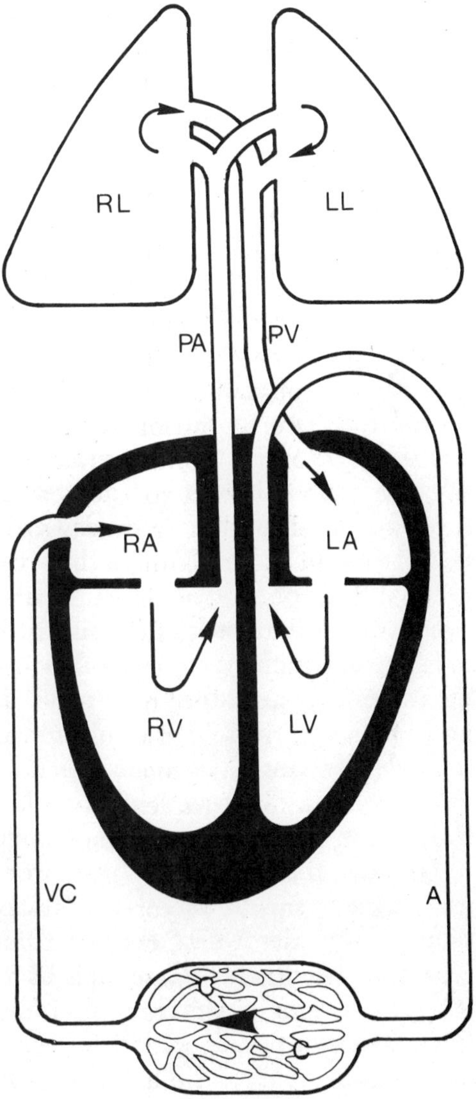

The cardiovascular system. Venous blood flows from the right ventricle (RV) into the pulmonary artery (PA), which carries it to the right and left lungs (RL and LL), where the blood is aerated. The oxygenated, or arterial, blood is carried via the pulmonary vein (PV) to the left auricle (LA) and thence the left ventricle (LV). The latter pumps the arterial blood into the aorta (A), which distributes it to the tissues through the capillaries (C). The used, or venous, blood is returned via the vena cava (VC) to the right auricle (RA) and back to the right ventricle to repeat the cycle.

ies, carrying oxygenated blood containing nutrients, are thick and strong, with a good deal of muscle in their walls to help propel the blood along. Veins, which return the used blood to the heart for repumping and recharging with oxygen and nutrients, are wider than the arteries but their walls are thinner (there is much less pressure within); they have fragile valves that keep the blood from flowing backward.

For some reason not well understood, certain molecules of lipid-protein complexes (primarily cholesterol) get into the tissues of artery walls but not, under normal circumstances, in those of the veins. This phenomenon may be the result of pressure, because if the blood pressure is elevated sufficiently within the veins for considerable time, deposits of lipoproteins can often be found in their walls. This is probably the reason why high blood pressure promotes and enhances atherosclerosis. Nonetheless, under ordinary circumstances atherosclerosis is a disease of arteries rather than veins.

I have stated that the complications of atherosclerosis kill over half our population. In this disease, complex combinations of fat collect in the walls of medium-size and large arteries. The presence of these materials destroys the continuity of the muscle and fibrous support of the vessel and so weakens the wall. It thickens the vessel wall, thereby narrowing the arterial channel, and finally it erodes the inner layers of the wall, causing a roughening of the lining surface. Wherever the vessel lining is roughened, the blood that flows over it is subjected to the clotting mechanism. A blood clot either obstructs the vessel or significantly narrows its channel. Damage to the arterial lining plus thickening and narrowing of the arterial walls, which diminishes vascular capacity, probably promote an elevation in the pressure of the blood within. In short, these conditions help bring about hypertension. Hypertension predisposes the vessel to a blowout or, by increasing the work load of the heart, leads to heart failure. By stretching and damaging the arterial walls, hypertension contributes to the depositing of fat complexes. We can say with a degree of certainty that hypertension worsens atherosclerosis and atherosclerosis worsens hypertension. Whatever the mechanism, the end result is a failure of the cir-

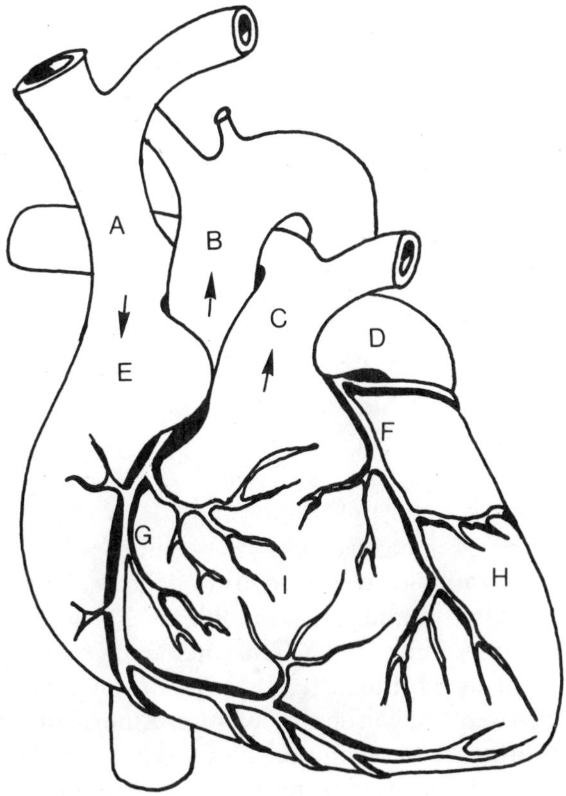

Exterior view of the heart from the front, showing the coronary blood vessels. (A) vena cava; (B) aorta; (C) pulmonary artery; (D) left auricle; (E) right auricle; (F) left coronary artery; (G) right coronary artery; (H) left ventricle; and (I) right ventricle.

culatory system to supply blood to a vital body part. The specific disease and its symptoms depend upon the vessel predominantly affected; and when all the diseases caused by atherosclerosis and hypertension are combined, they add up to an appalling figure. There is no other health hazard to compare with it. Every sensible person should strive to learn as much as he can about this menace. Much of this book is devoted to a simple explanation of what is known about this disease and how we may be able to prevent it.

3

Atherosclerosis, the Killer

It causes, or helps to cause, more than half of all deaths in the industrialized countries of the world. Atherosclerosis is older than the Egyptian mummies. Its incidence has increased more than fifteen times since 1920. This incidence can almost certainly be reduced significantly, perhaps dramatically, by simple dietary precautions. Yet the average American is ignorant of this condition and its importance. When his attention is called to this extraordinary disease, he mumbles, "Ah yes, hardening of the arteries; I can't do anything about that, can I?"

He not only can; he jolly well better!

The public knows so little about atherosclerosis because when grandpa departed this world at age seventy-three, the doctor said a stroke had carried him off. When his wife died some years later (she had experienced mental deterioration for six years), the doctor wrote "senility" on the death certificate. Even when Uncle Willy died of a heart attack, no one mentioned the word *atherosclerosis;* yet atherosclerosis was the root of all these troubles (cerebrovascular accident, senile dementia, and myocardial infarction), and death might have been prevented or at least delayed had the family taken a few simple and sensible dietary precautions.

It is high time that we all familiarize ourselves with the facts and more probable theories about this matter.

Atherosclerosis is a degenerative disease of our large and medium-size arteries. It is a cumulative disease that probably begins in infancy and reaches a stage detectable (by a physician) by about forty years of age. It causes arteries to decay in focal areas, and in one way or another the lesions interfere with the passage of blood through the affected arteries. The tissues normally supplied are deprived of oxygen and nourishment. The symptoms of atherosclerosis do not appear until actual vessel obstruction occurs, and these symptoms will be as varied as are the arteries affected. The average layperson would have no reason to suppose that stroke, heart attack, and gangrene of the big toe are all caused by the same generic disease, atherosclerosis.

The Greeks supply us with its name: *athēra* ("gruel") and *sklēros* ("hard"). It is not a very appropriate term, because only a few of the lesions are filled with a porridgelike material; the plaque, unless it is calcified, is apt to be softer than normal tissue. The first recorded description of the lesion is probably that of Leonardo da Vinci in the fifteenth century. Leonardo had an insatiable curiosity about everything, and nothing was too sacred to stay his inquisitive probe. Three centuries later, Rudolf Virchow, known as the father of pathology, gave the first theory of its mechanism. Virchow believed that the lesion of atherosclerosis was caused by an infiltration of fatty substances from the blood into the arterial wall. The matter has been a major topic of argument among research workers in the health field ever since.

The characteristic lesion of atherosclerosis seems to be caused by an interference in the routine life processes of certain cells in the innermost layer (intima) of arteries. Taken as a group, the chemical activities of a cell are called its metabolism. Intracellular metabolism is so complicated that we need not involve ourselves in its complexities; we will use the term to indicate processes, even though the details are not germane to our discussion.

As I have already suggested, man is a carnivore (meat-eater) only by adaptation. Among the foods for which he was designed to eat were a number of vegetable fats, all unsaturated with hydrogen. We say that fats are saturated when their chemical bonds, instead of remaining free, are attached to other atoms, often hydrogen. Early man's metabolic machinery was able to handle the unsaturated fats efficiently but unequipped to metabolize the saturated ones. Eve's apple was probably not an apple at all; more likely it was a plump little hamster that the old serpent had snared and brought up to her tree house. She apparently enjoyed the repast but probably suffered from dyspepsia afterward because animal fats differ from vegetable fats. They are more saturated and man's metabolic equipment was not intended to handle them. Although the food must certainly have been more interesting than the accustomed vegetarian fare, things were never the same again about the house.

In one way or another, fatty substances from animal fats seeped into the intima of the arterial walls. They permeated the lining, especially at points where it had been injured, as in those areas where the intima had been stretched and battered by excessive pressures. Given a few million years, nature designed a protective mechanism that could clean up the fatty debris that defaced arterial walls. She modified the metabolic habits of certain cells (scavenger cells) of the vessel wall so they could gobble up the unwanted fat and carry it away to the liver, the main waste-processing plant. But only a limited amount could be handled in this manner, and the system was not very efficient. Minute deposits of lipid can be found deposited in points and streaks in the aortas of infants less than a year old. The drama of atherosclerosis probably follows, more or less faithfully, the synopsis given below.

Lipids seep out of the blood and into the linings of the arteries. They do this especially in areas where the lining is subject to injury: at the beginning of the aorta, in the first third of the arteries that supply the heart (coronary arteries), in the vessels of the brain and kidneys, and in the arteries of the lower extremities where, because the columns of blood hang downward, the pressure is greatest.

It has recently become apparent that when there is an increase in the amount of certain types of lipids in the blood, there is a greater tendency for seepage of these materials into

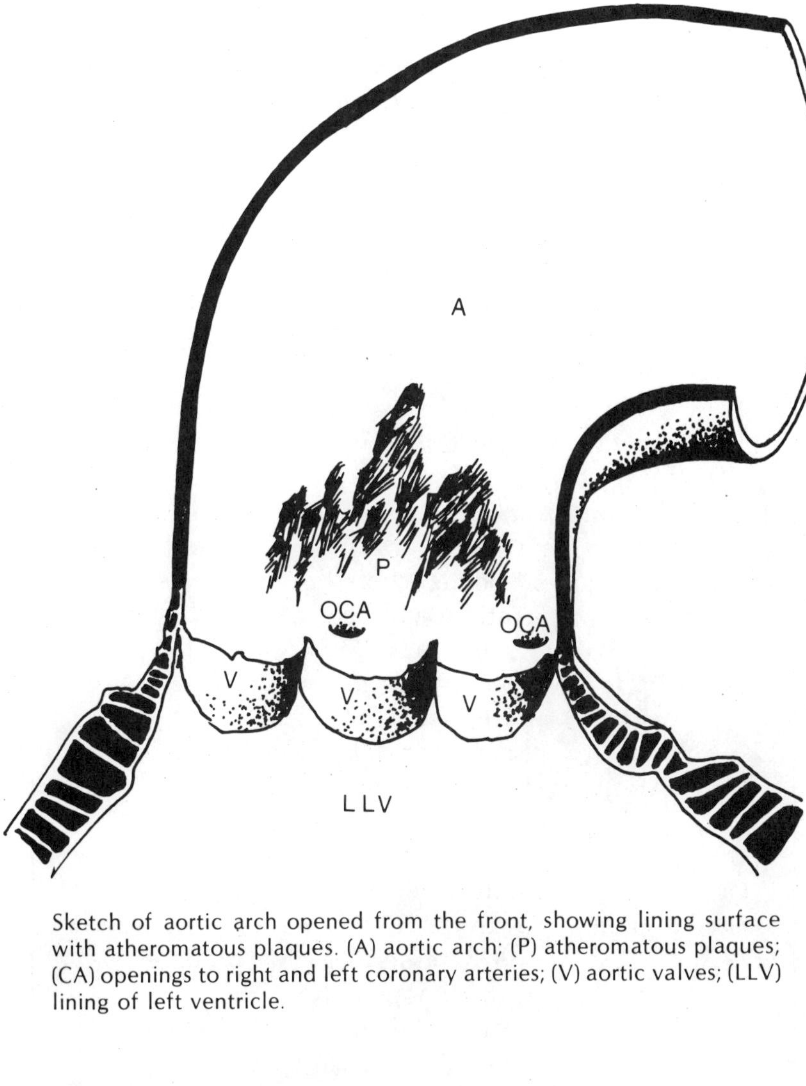

Sketch of aortic arch opened from the front, showing lining surface with atheromatous plaques. (A) aortic arch; (P) atheromatous plaques; (CA) openings to right and left coronary arteries; (V) aortic valves; (LLV) lining of left ventricle.

the vessel walls. These mechanisms will be discussed in Chapter 4, where the causes of atherosclerosis are examined.

When the amount of lipid in the arterial walls is greater than can be cleaned up by the scavenger cells, it begins to pile up. The abnormal accumulations interfere with the normal metabolic activities of the resident cells. If the latter are surrounded

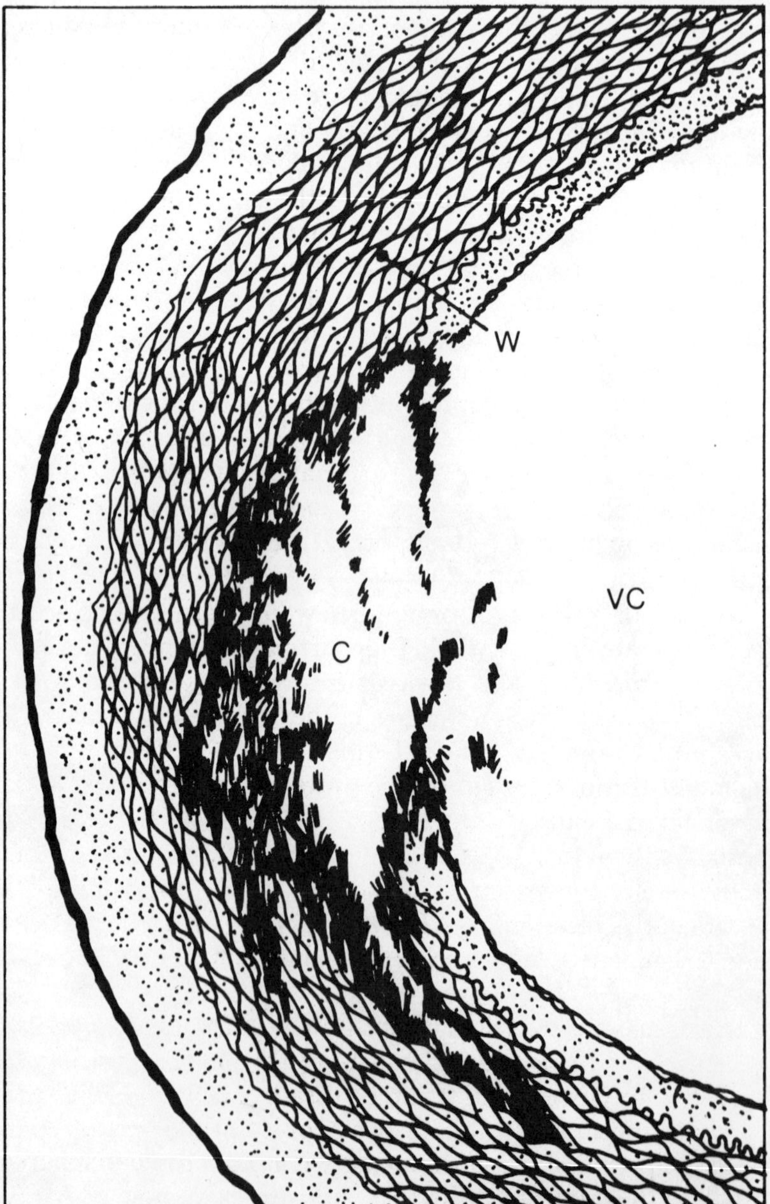

Cross section of an arterial segment. An atheromatous plaque has formed in the wall. It is splitting the wall into layers and has ruptured into the arterial channel. The dark granules in the plaque are crystals of calcium salts. (VC) vessel channel; (C) channel in aneurysm; (W) wall of artery.

by a coating of fat, they cannot absorb their quota of nourishment and oxygen, nor expel carbon dioxide and other wastes. They languish and die, adding more unwanted debris to the pile. Lymph pathways are blocked and fluid accumulates, a condition called edema. The mass of cells increases in size. Sooner or later a tiny blood vessel within the arterial wall ruptures and blood escapes into the lesion, adding more litter and increasing the pressure within the damaged area. The walls of this lesion erode into the central cavity that has been formed, and the area of destruction enlarges. It extends into the middle layer of the arterial wall and eventually breaks through the lining and discharges its semiliquid, fatty, gruellike contents into the blood stream.

The lining membrane of the arterial channel is now broken; its surface is no longer perfectly smooth. When this happens, the door is open for a very important and dangerous complication.

Millions of years ago, organisms were doomed to bleed to death whenever an opening occurred in their circulatory systems. Nature devised a way to prevent this hazard. When blood flows over a rough surface, eddies occur at the margins of the current and the rate of flow decreases. When blood stagnates, fibrin, a tough, elastic protein, is precipitated out of the blood and causes a clot. Blood also clots when it comes in contact with injured tissue, which contains a substance that promotes clot formation. A blood clot, or thrombus, forms at the site of the vessel injury. The network of fibrin catches blood cells and platelets, and a solid thrombus is built on the wall of the vessel.

This is all very well if there is a hole to be plugged to prevent the escape of blood, the reason why the clotting mechanism evolved in the first place. It can be disastrous, however, if there is no hole and the thrombus grows to obstruct the arterial channel. That is exactly what happens in coronary thrombosis (coronary occlusion, heart attack) and many cases of stroke (cerebrovascular accident).

Abnormal deposits of certain lipids within tissue cause calcium salts in the blood stream to precipitate out and deposit themselves in the fatty lesion. The lipid becomes encrusted with crystalline calcium deposits. This portion of the vessel becomes rigid and as hard and brittle as chalk. Further, craggy masses exaggerate the roughness of the plaque and encourage additional thrombus formation. Calcium salts are much less permeable to x-rays than normal tissue is, so calcified plaques can be identified on x-ray films of patients suspected of severe atherosclerosis.

The atheromatous lesion often ruptures into the vessel channel, but it may also extend more deeply into the wall. As the buildup progresses, the vessel wall becomes weaker at this point. One of three things is apt to happen. The excavation may perforate the outer wall and cause profuse bleeding into body tissues; if the accident occurs near a natural body space such as the chest or abdominal cavity, internal bleeding, to the point of death, may occur without a drop of blood apparent on the exterior; or third, the wall may be weakened to such an extent that the outer layers are stretched like a balloon. An immense blood-filled sac may form and press against vital organs such as the lungs or the heart, interfering with their function. This lesion is called an aneurysm. The most common complication is a variation of this: the cavity extends outward, the pressure of the blood within splits the layers of the arterial wall, and long extensions are formed under hydraulic pressure for great distances along the vessel. This is called a dissecting aneurysm. Perforations and aneurysms are almost entirely limited to the aorta, the great artery that leads from the heart, and thus occur within the chest or abdomen.

It is apparent that the symptoms of atheromatous lesions depend upon their site in the affected artery. The first portion of the aorta as it emerges from the heart is the part usually affected. It is rare to encounter an aorta in anyone forty years or older that is not scarred by at least some atheromatous deposits. Because the aorta is the largest artery in the body, its channel is not so likely to be obstructed by a thrombus as a medium-size artery is. The arteries most commonly involved are the two that supply the heart muscle. This, of course, is a catastrophe, because the heart muscle needs a constant and abundant supply of fresh blood for its work, and life is totally dependent upon its continuous function. For that reason, coronary occlusion is the most common and most lethal type of atherosclerosis.

Earlier writers of medical texts referred to degenerative diseases of the arteries as arteriosclerosis. Before long it became apparent that there are two important types of arteriosclerosis. The most prevalent of these, which we have just described, affects large- and medium-size arteries and is caused by the formation of atheromatous plaques. This is called atherosclerosis. A second variety, less common, affects the small arteries and is essentially a thickening of the middle layer (media) of their walls. Although it is frequently accompanied by atheromatous plaques, it was recognized as a separate entity and named arteriolarsclerosis (small arteries are called arterioles). Then it was learned that arteriolarsclerosis made one more likely to develop atherosclerosis and accelerated the progress of the disease, and atherosclerosis, in turn, seemed to have a similar effect on arteriolarsclerosis. The outstanding clinical feature of arteriolarsclerosis is high blood pressure; this condition is not encountered in uncomplicated atherosclerosis. Both types of arteriosclerosis, alone or together, are responsible for the second most common cause of cardiovascular death, stroke (cerebrovascular accident or CVA).

Another disease associated with atherosclerosis, senile dementia, is the result of lack of sufficient blood supply to the brain to maintain it in a healthy state. It begins about twenty-five years later than atherosclerotic heart disease. One reason for the age difference is that the carotid artery, which brings blood to the brain, is larger than the coronary arteries and thus takes longer to become clogged. A second reason, when the smaller intracerebral arteries are involved, is that the brain simply has more blood vessels than the heart and so a greater number of vessels must be involved before problems begin to show up.

Atherosclerosis may affect the heart itself or the aorta. When it affects the heart, the valves stiffen as the result of calcium deposits in the atheromatous plaques. The valves either do not close completely or the stony masses obstruct the blood flow through the valve openings. Both types can cause eventual heart failure because either a leaking or obstructed valve means additional work for the heart. When atherosclerosis affects the wall of the aorta, it may partially obstruct the channels of the large arteries that supply blood to the legs; it may also produce massive deposits of cholesterol in the wall of the aorta itself.

When the arteries of the arms and legs are affected by atherosclerosis, the resulting condition is called peripheral vascular disease. At first, the decreased blood supply causes muscle cramps and episodes of tingling in the fingers or toes. Ability to exercise is drastically limited; sometimes the victim can be up and about for as little as half an hour before having to rest. In a severe form the affected limb may turn blue (cyanotic), especially when cold, because the used blood is not replaced quickly enough and the tissues lack sufficient oxygen. The worst stage is complete arterial occlusion and gangrene of the affected part, at which point amputation may be necessary.

Although atherosclerosis causes other diseases, which vary depending upon the vessels predominantly affected, these are not, as a group, as numerically important as any one of the conditions we have discussed. Clearly, the related diseases of atherosclerosis and hypertension constitute the most important health hazard of our time. If anything can be done to prevent these disorders, we should certainly do it.

The medical profession may not completely understand the mechanisms of atherosclerosis, but the American people are beginning to recognize its importance. Anything that will help increase public knowledge of it should be favorably considered.

From the preceding discussion it is clear that the term atherosclerosis has been a sleeper, an alligator densely shrouded in a scientific terminology that invites ennui rather than concern. I have described the lesions of this ubiquitous disease in some detail because I am certain that each of you has this condition to some degree and that it is measuring the days of your life as surely as does the watch on your wrist. It seems sensible to insist that we all know at least as much about something that may take our lives as we do about our timepieces.

4

The Causes of Atherosclerosis

Nature has done her best to insure our bodies a safe and satisfactory food supply. She has provided us with a double set of taste organs, the olfactory bulbs in our noses and the taste buds on our tongues, a setup that long ago was programed, albeit not very effectively, for the broad distinction between good and evil. This system rewards us with a sensation of pleasure when it encounters food it considers healthy and it warns us with a bad taste if the food seems injurious or dubious. It is an ancient mechanism shared by most living things. Even the unicellular animals exhibit positive and negative reactions to helpful and harmful environmental substances.

The system has numerous weaknesses. With the use of his sense of taste alone, man is often unable to tell the difference between edible mushrooms and poisonous toadstools, whereas some animals can apparently make this distinction without cerebral effort. For most immediate and catastrophic dangers, however, the system works fairly well. That is, it works the way nature intended it to work: it helps protect us from the noxious agents that might cause sudden death. Paradoxically, it aids and abets our worst enemy, atherosclerosis. It does so by offering us a pleasurable experience when tasting the elements that carry most of food's flavor, the lure for eating. These are the fats.

Because the lethal effects of atherosclerosis begin in the mid-forties, the end of the reproductive period, it is quite clear what nature has been up to. She has done a fairly efficient job of protecting us through the early period, which she considers so important. There is no question but that she is fixated on reproduction. She programed *Homo sapiens* to get the job done by the onset of menopause; after that the poor old thing must look to him or herself for survival. Nature's plan can hardly be considered far-sighted for the good of the world of people; her plans rarely are. At this point in our history she has handed us a real dilemma and left us to deal with it ourselves. Unaltered, the world's present birth rate could lead to population growth that would be catastrophic by the end of the century. That is the way nature works—a minor error here, a whopper there; who cares about catastrophes as long as the seed is saved?

Nature and man are in sharp disagreement about the matter of longevity. Our taste system provides us with protection only through the first half of our lives; then atherosclerosis sets in. Small wonder that man has taken an attitude somewhat different from that of nature. Worse, he was slow in catching on. Not until about half a century ago did he come to realize the full menace of atherosclerosis. Even today he does not understand this metabolic aberration fully, but he is making a heroic attempt to do so. Within a decade or two he will have the formulas worked out. Nonetheless, there are some of us who cannot wait. Atherosclerosis is a cumulative alteration of the arteries. Once the vessels are affected, the damage probably can never be repaired. It behooves each of us to do what he or she can now. Let us review the facts as we see them.

There are two key aspects in the consideration of a diet that will promote optimum health. First, our bodies can utilize only a limited number of calories in their energy expenditure. If the amount ingested is greater than the amount spent, the excess must be stored. A limited store of reserve energy is essential in order to keep metabolic processes constant, but excessive collections of stored fats tax the heart and interfere with the function of other vital organs. Because nature has failed at this task, the body requires help to balance the getting and spending of energy. We have to recognize a fundamental law. Gross obesity is not common in the wild state. When food supplies are too abundant for the population to use up, the population will increase until a balance is achieved. In short, the living organism is programed for a lean diet. Food consumption in greater amounts than can be used for energy needs leads to obesity, a disturbance in vital physiology.

The second dietary factor to consider is that ingestion of fats that cannot be completely utilized leads to arterial disease. The history of this finding constitutes one of the most complicated accounts in medical history.

It was almost fifty years ago that physicians noticed that people with high blood-cholesterol levels were more apt to die of atherosclerosis than those whose levels were normal. It was quite reasonable to conclude that those who ate large amounts of cholesterol should have high levels of cholesterol in their blood. Then someone spoiled this easy conclusion by showing that a stable blood-cholesterol level could be maintained even though no cholesterol was ingested. The body apparently makes its own.

"Ah yes," came the rebuttal. "The body can make cholesterol, but it makes excess cholesterol only when an excess of fats is ingested."

"But what about the Italians? They live on olive oil and there is no great preponderance of atherosclerosis in Italy."

"Ah, but it is not just the amount of fat that is eaten; it is its quality, its degree of saturation. Olive oil is of vegetable origin, relatively unsaturated and therefore less apt to cause atherosclerosis."

"But what about Eskimos? Seal blubber is not a vegetable fat."

"No, but seal blubber is one of the few animal fats that is relatively unsaturated."

And so the argument progressed over the years. I was reminded that I had drunk whole milk all through my youth, lots of it and the richer the better. Then, shortly out of medical school, I encountered a youngster, age fourteen, dead from atherosclerotic coronary occlusion. His coronary arteries looked like those I was seeing in patients in their forties. This boy had an interesting history. Arty had been struck down by poliomyelitis at the age of six. His thoracic muscles were paralyzed and for eight years he had lived in an iron lung. He was a nice-looking chap with a wonderful personality. He never complained. Everyone who knew him came to love him—nurses, doctors, all the visitors to his fellow patients on the ward. Everyone wanted to do something nice for Arty, but there isn't much one can do for a boy who must spend his entire day and all his nights in a cylinder of steel with his head protruding through a hole in a heavy rubber diaphragm. But Arty liked ice cream, and everyone brought him ice cream—quarts of it, every day—and Arty ate it. For nearly eight years he ate ice cream and took no exercise whatsoever. It takes a person with a normal exercise routine and an ordinary food intake about thirty years to accumulate sufficient atheromatous plaques to close his left coronary artery. It took Arty only eight.

At about the same time, a group of army physicians published an interesting report on the incidence of coronary occlusion among draftees serving in Korea. The Korean War was peculiar in more than one respect. It was a limited war fought during good times. The civilian population in the United States had plenty of everything and wanted their soldiers to have plenty of everything, too, everything that might ease their burden of hardship and loneliness. Ice cream was a small thing to provide—ice cream, marbleized steaks, butter, and lots of nice rich milk. Enough of these foods was provided for every soldier every time he felt like having some. It was a small thing, to be sure, but it was enough to fill our soldiers' hearts with gratitude and atheromatous plaques, or so concluded the physicians who made a survey concerning the relationship of a fatty diet and coronary artery disease.

Some years later, a friend of mine, a prominent heart specialist and later president of the American College of Physicians, visited a large civilian hospital in Tokyo. He was shown through ward after ward, each with a hundred or more interesting cases of everything except coronary occlusion, that type of heart disease in which the arteries that supply the heart muscle are corroded with atherosclerotic plaques.

"Now show me your coronary ward," requested my friend.

"But we don't have one," his hosts replied. "There aren't enough heart attacks here to fill a ward."

The explanation lies, no doubt, in the low fat content of the Japanese diet. If Oriental food is characterized by the parsimonious use of fat, the Western diet is its antithesis. We are inclined to judge the merit of our dishes by the degree of their richness; that is, by their shortening or fat content. We are conditioned to the association of fat and flavor; the two are synonymous. If one egg makes a dish taste rich, then three eggs should make it taste absolutely scrumptious. We relish desserts such as those made exclusively of butter, chocolate, and sugar. They are delicious and rich—rich and lethal. Our own Southern cooking is apt to employ large amounts of fats in its recipes. The story is told of the Southern cook who comes into the kitchen, sets out on the mixing table a bowl of eggs, a crock of butter, a pitcher of cream, and a pail of lard and then asks, "Now let's see, what shall I make today?"

I have a friend, a doctor, who is fully cognizant of the importance of dietary discretion. He has a large family. When I last talked with him a few years ago, his children knew almost nothing of the forbidden fats because these items were simply not allowed in the family kitchen. It will be interesting to learn, years hence, when the children have left the family environment and are free to eat what they choose, if they will have developed a distaste for what we now believe to be the high-risk lipid diet. It will also be interesting to note among those who remain faithful to the family precepts what the incidence of atherosclerosis is. I suspect that it will be rewardingly low.

An analysis of atheromatous plaque in the vessel wall shows it to be composed of cholesterol-ester complexes. Originally it was thought that cholesterol was the mischief maker, and physicians sought to reduce the blood level of this specific substance by limiting its dietary intake. It was a time when egg yolks fell into disfavor and vegetable oils began to replace butter in many diets. We found out that it wasn't that simple. Cholesterol is necessary in normal cell metabolism; if the diet doesn't supply it the tissue will make it. The cholesterol levels of most people may be controlled by limiting the intake of cholesterol and the materials of which cholesterol is made, the saturated fats. For a period we became a nation dedicated to the elimination of saturated fats as food components, and again we had to learn that it isn't even that simple.

Cholesterol is a lipid complex. It rarely occurs in a pure form in our metabolic routines. Instead, most of it is bound in complicated chains with protein components; these chains are called lipoproteins. They are categorized according to the relative densities of lipid and protein, measured by means of a centrifuge. When a test tube of fluid is spun in a centrifuge, a simple device that is little more than a rapidly spinning wheel, the contents are separated into their component parts, which are in turn forced to the bottom of the test tube in layers by order of their density. In the case of fat and protein compounds, the proteins, being the largest molecules, form one layer. The proteins combined with about a 25 percent lipid form another layer. These are called high-density lipoproteins or HDLs. Proteins with a 75 percent lipid component form the third layer and are called low-density lipoproteins or LDLs.

It has been known for some time that in people with high levels of HDL in their blood, coronary occlusion and atherosclerosis are unusual; those with low HDL levels and high LDL levels have a high incidence of these conditions. This may seem unnecessarily complicated and contradictory at first reading, but it is neither. Instead, it is a simple and concise explanation for atherosclerosis. It is concluded that high levels of HDL protect against formation of atherosclerotic plaques. Furthermore, it has been found that low-saturated-fat diets will lower LDL levels experimentally in animals; but when early experimentation indicated that low-saturated-fat diets decreased HDL levels as well, an alarm was sent out that people on these diets might be unwittingly increasing their chances of developing coronary disease. It now seems that at least some HDL is derived from LDL, which is why a decrease in the latter tends to decrease the former. The important point is that lower levels of LDL tend to mean lower incidence of atherosclerosis.

All of this sounds logical enough; the facts are there, the conclusions obvious. High dietary intake of animal fat results in high levels of cholesterol in the LDL factor of blood lipoproteins. People with high levels of LDL have much more atherosclerosis than do those with low levels. Ergo, high LDL levels cause atherosclerosis. Let's get on with the job and eradicate animal fats from the diet. Next question, please.

But again, the matter is not that simple. A number of convincing studies indicate that elimination of saturated fat from the diet, even for as long as five years, does not decrease the incidence of death from coronary artery disease. The statistics are all there, but we cannot nail down the conclusion experimentally, probably because it is still too early.

A recent report, May, 1980, by the Food and Nutrition Board of the National Research Council has created considerable dismay among United States health professionals and confusion with the public. The board stated, in essence, that it found no statistical evidence that reducing blood levels of cholesterol by dietary methods prevented coronary heart disease. The report is completely honest, but the board apparently assumed that the public would be able to interpret its conclusion realistically.

The predictable result is that one commonly hears the following complaint among laypeople: "Why can't the doctors make up their minds? First they told us not to eat saturated fats and now they say eat as much cholesterol as you like."

This is almost certainly not the conclusion that the board intended the public to draw. The report should have stated that atherosclerosis is a cumulative condition that starts at birth and reaches its peak, in the majority of cases, after the age of forty-five. Conclusions based on statistics gathered from experiments in which reduced fat intake was maintained over shorter periods cannot be considered valid. To stress these and ignore the vast amount of epidemiologic data that have been gathered around the world over the past half century could set back medical progress and result in incalculable numbers of unnecessary coronary-related deaths.

It is reasonable to suggest that human diets are too hard to control and that atherosclerosis is a cumulative disease. Perhaps it takes all of the first forty years that man usually lives on his fatty diet to produce the plaques that cause death. Perhaps, but there are some other disturbing data, data that will not go away when we turn our backs.

It has been shown that certain types of protein raise the

cholesterol levels in animals. For example, diets high in casein, the protein found in milk and cheese, will cause excessive amounts of cholesterol in the blood of rabbits. On the other hand, other types of protein, soybean protein for example, tend to lower cholesterol levels. It appears that animal proteins are bad and plant proteins, such as those from peas, sunflower seeds, and soybeans, are good. In short, some researchers insist that animal protein raises cholesterol levels.

There are other complications to harass our credibility: a high intake of certain simple sugars such as fructose and sucrose make high cholesterol levels even higher while the more complicated polysaccharides (starches and cellulose) do just the opposite.

Some recent work reveals that certain trace metals, specifically copper and zinc, may be related to the problem. It seems to be a matter of their ratio. High copper–low zinc levels tend to keep the cholesterol content down; the reverse allows it to rise.

All of this is related to the high level of cholesterol in the bloodstream, but some theorists point out that cholesterol (in the LDL form) is not the only lipid in blood serum. They insist that there are other factors that seem to be related to atherosclerosis. These are the triglycerides. Beautiful charts can be drawn related to these substances, suggesting that triglycerides are as damaging as LDL.

I have given this briefest of summaries of atherosclerosis research in an attempt to present you with a fair picture. It is obvious that the matter is far from settled. The evidence against animal fat is overwhelming and undisputed, but it is based on epidemiological observation and that can be tenuous. This type of data, garnered from the study and comparison of statistics concerning various national, regional, racial, or social populations, is sometimes more convincing than warranted. It certainly is true that people with high cholesterol levels have an increased incidence of atherosclerosis and that these levels can be reduced by removing animal fat from the diet. What we lack is conclusive statistical proof. Then what is the poor, confused layperson to do?

First, we must maintain an open mind and test all possibilities. Next, we should formulate a concept of atherosclerosis that will allow us to consider a number of factors in its cause. And finally, because it may be decades before a universally satisfactory resolution is reached, we must use the best knowledge that is currently available. We have to adjust our diets to the most reasonable compromise. Our food intake should be low in animal fat and palm, coconut, and peanut oils; it must contain as little casein (most cheeses are very rich in casein) and as much plant protein as possible. Our intake of sugars should veer to the side of the complex polysaccharides (vegetables and starches) and away from the simpler monosaccharides (refined sugar). Some day we might even have to readjust our copper-zinc ratio to acceptable levels by means of pills, just as we supplement our daily vitamin intake.

We should certainly keep our total caloric intake down to maintain our weight a bit under that suggested by the standard tables. We should understand the energy balance and we should exercise to the maximum of common sense and good judgment. And last, we should start all of these programs early, probably in childhood. For those of us too old for that, there is no better time than the present.

It would seem that man has evolved from the lower forms as a herbivorous animal. His metabolic system was genetically programed to metabolize large amounts of fibrous carbohydrates with essential vegetable proteins and almost no fat. He had to synthesize most of the necessary lipids from the polysaccharides he gathered from the plant world. He eventually mixed in a few insects with his leaves, berries, and nuts, and found them agreeable. Small animals, rodents, reptiles, and birds were plentiful, so he conditioned his palate to his supply potential, and soon established the society recognized by anthropologists as hunters and gatherers. In time he became omnivorous and acquired a fancy for the flavors that fats impart.

However, cells cannot change their genetic constituents to match the habits of their hosts. They go right on replicating themselves century after century, frozen in their genetic choreography until a mistake, a breach of natural law, produces a change in the spatial relationship of the molecules that compose their genetic apparatus. The great majority of these mistakes come to no good; the organisms that are the unfortunate bearers are usually defective and die without progeny. But once in a while the accidental change is for the better. The recipient is more capable and more successful at life and reproduction than his brethren. He survives and reproduces and his progeny start a new and stronger race.

Our venerable ancestor (probably *Australopithecus*) adapted himself to the metabolic routines of a carnivore. But he had the same old cells, and cells cannot forget; he was still a herbivore, but now one with exotic tastes. He was called an omnivore, but his cells were a bit clumsy in handling the fats that they were forced to process. Incomplete metabolic products of the animal fats he ingested cluttered his blood stream and began to corrode his arteries. His new habits had given him atherosclerosis, a curse visited upon his children. But nature didn't care. "Get your reproduction work done early," she advised, "and history won't mind."

Perhaps history doesn't mind, but you and I do. We have to take charge, change our taste preferences, and keep things on the right course. In order to do that we must understand the relation of diet to health and longevity. The remainder of this book is concerned with the diseases caused by poor diet and exercise habits. In the following chapter we shall consider the most important of these.

5

Myocardial Infarction

Myocardial infarction, sometimes called coronary occlusion or coronary thrombosis or, in lay terms, heart attack, is the most common cause of death in all males over the age of thirty-five; it is the most common cause of death in both males and females over forty-five. This condition strikes males between the ages of thirty-five and forty-five about five times as often as it does females of the same age. It appears, therefore, that females are usually spared until after menopause. Nature has little sympathy for the female who can no longer bear children, and she eventually becomes just as vulnerable as a man; her rate of accumulation of atherosclerotic plaques speeds up in later life. It is interesting to note in this connection that giving estrogen, the female sex hormone, decreases the amount of low-density lipoprotein (LDL) in the blood, whereas androgen, the male sex hormone, increases it.

The incidence of coronary heart disease in blacks, both male and female, is higher at all ages than in whites. The reason seems to be associated with the higher incidence of hypertension among blacks. Blacks who die of myocardial infarction usually have severely high blood pressure. I know of no reason other than a genetic one to explain this.

There are other types of heart disease, but none can compare in frequency and deadliness to coronary heart disease. Congenital heart disease (abnormal development of the heart while the fetus is in the uterus) is the most important of these. A considerable proportion of such cases can now be treated surgically.

A type of heart disease that was once more common than myocardial infarction occurs in the heart that is scarred as a result of rheumatic fever. That disease, once dreaded as the killer of children and young adults, is caused by an allergy to the toxins of certain bacteria. It results in inflammation of the arterial linings. About 3 percent of those with strep throat (a precursor of rheumatic fever) will develop heart disease. In about 50 percent of children who have had obvious rheumatic fever, the covering layers of the heart valves will become inflamed. After the inflammation subsides, scars remain. Over a period of years the valves become distorted by these scars until they no longer function properly. Rheumatic heart disease manifests itself a few months after the acute episode of the rheumatic fever that initiated it; heart failure comes on many years later because of the scarring of the valves. Rheumatic fever is rare nowadays because the bacteria that cause it can be effectively combatted with antibiotics. The cardiac complications are, therefore, most unusual because the disease can be treated before it has a chance to affect the heart.

Other microorganisms can damage the heart. In the past, the most fearsome infection was subacute bacterial endocarditis, but now this can usually be controlled with antibiotics, as can the spirochete of syphilis, another culprit causing heart infection. The result is that the cardiac manifestations of these conditions are unusual where health care is adequate.

When one of the coronary arteries becomes effectively narrowed by atherosclerosis or completely obstructed by a thrombus (blood clot), the portion of the muscle supplied by that artery is deprived of its supply of oxygen. Muscle cells, both cardiac and voluntary (such as those of our arms and legs), differ from other body cells in that they can go into oxygen debt. When the supply of oxygen to these cells is insufficient, they are able to burn parts of themselves for a short period of time in order to continue functioning. Nonetheless, the normal metabolic process cannot be completed under these circumstances, and lactic acid accumulates within the cell. When a certain

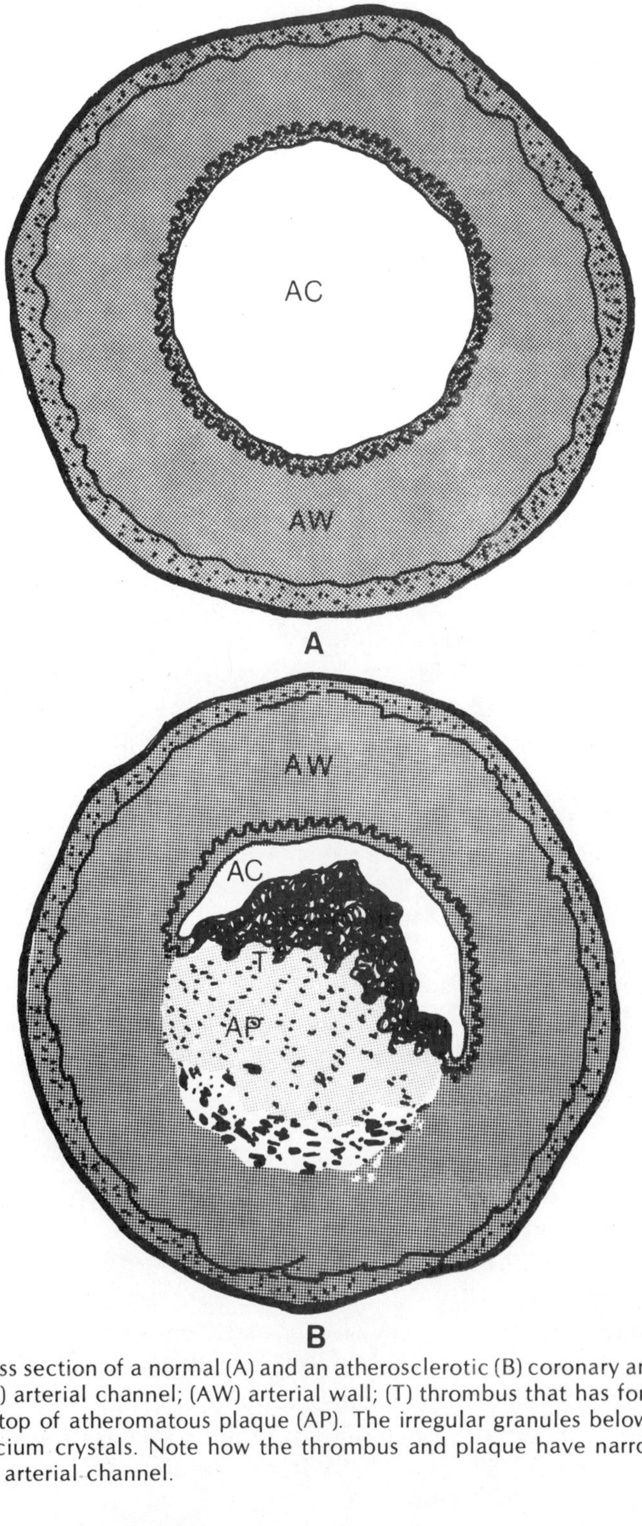

Cross section of a normal (A) and an atherosclerotic (B) coronary artery. (AC) arterial channel; (AW) arterial wall; (T) thrombus that has formed on top of atheromatous plaque (AP). The irregular granules below are calcium crystals. Note how the thrombus and plaque have narrowed the arterial channel.

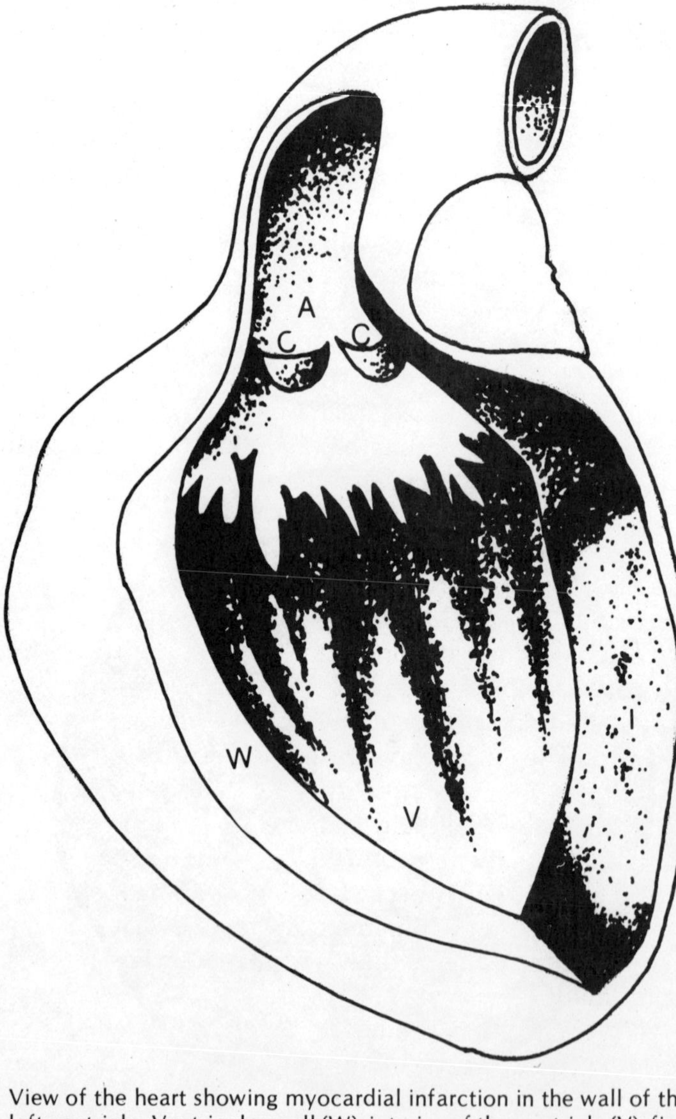

View of the heart showing myocardial infarction in the wall of the left ventricle. Ventricular wall (W); interior of the ventricle (V); first portion of the aortic arch (A): (C) aortic valves; (I) infarct (area of muscle degeneration). This lesion is the result of an occlusion of the left coronary artery.

level of lactic acid has been reached, the cell is poisoned and dies. This is what happens when a coronary artery is blocked by a thrombus. The aggregate of cells that are affected produces a dead area called an infarct. Myocardial (heart muscle) infarction is the technical name for heart attack.

Many kinds of body cells are replaced by their neighboring cells when they die. Skin cells normally die and slough off with the result that the epidermis is changed every few days. The lining cells of the gastrointestinal tract are even more ephemeral. Some blood cells live for only a few hours. All these cells are replaced periodically by new, young cells that carry on the functions of the old ones. But muscle cells, alas, do not have this proclivity. They make a feeble attempt at replication, but the new cells never reach maturity and functional efficiency. An infarct of the heart is an area of dead muscle that cannot contract and, even worse, may be ruptured by the blood under pressure within the heart chambers when the remaining healthy muscle contracts.

The diagnosis of myocardial infarction is not always obvious to the layperson. In the first hours, many of its victims believe they are having an attack of indigestion, even though the typical symptom is sudden intense pain in the center of the chest. Most victims describe their pain as the worst they have ever suffered, so severe that they are forced to stop what they are doing and lie down. They often have the sensation of being strangled. Most describe the pain as "squeezing" or "crushing." In about a quarter of the cases this pain radiates to the arms, more frequently to the left arm. Sometimes it extends into the neck and jaw or to the abdomen or back. In many cases the pain is much less severe, and in about 15 percent of the cases there is no pain at all. It is in these patients that an erroneous diagnosis is most frequently made.

The pain comes from the heart muscle itself, when the demand for oxygen is greater than the supply. Because there are other conditions in which this situation applies, the occurence of chest pain does not necessarily spell myocardial infarction.

The heart is supplied with blood by the right and left coronary arteries, which branch off the aorta just after it emerges from the heart. If the pressure within the aorta falls to a level that is inadequate to fill the coronary arteries—or if the oxygen level within the blood falls to a critical level for reasons entirely unrelated to the cardiovascular system—the heart muscle is plunged into a state of oxygen deprivation, and pain is the result. When a portion of the heart is infarcted, its contraction may be so severely impaired that the blood pressure falls to a level at which the uninvolved muscle cells cannot receive sufficient oxygen for proper function. This sets off a vicious, often fatal, cycle.

There are mechanisms other than myocardial infarction that create an oxygen deficit and consequent cardiac pain. If you increase the demand for oxygen by exercise, or by walking against a wind (particularly a cold wind), or even by exposure to an intense emotional experience, and if your heart is operating at the time with marginal efficiency, heart pain may result. Such pain, when caused by anything other than infarction, is called angina pectoris or just angina (from the Greek word for strangling).

You doubtless know people who have had severe angina pectoris. Attacks of angina are more apt to be precipitated in the morning, before the patient gets "warmed up," than at other times of the day. Sometimes it takes nothing more than a few stairs, a short burst of anger, or even the minor exertion of shaving to bring on the attack. The pain of angina pectoris is severe but rarely as bad as that of myocardial infarction; it ceases spontaneously after a few minutes and is completely relieved by nitroglycerin, which causes dilation of the involved artery and thus allows more blood to flow through. The pain of myocardial infarction persists and cannot be relieved by medication. Further, it occurs only once for each infarct, whereas a person may experience literally thousands of angina attacks.

Atheromatous plaques within the coronary arteries make one more likely to experience anginal pain. It is also true that people with atherosclerosis (and angina pectoris) are more prone to myocardial infarction. Nonetheless, a distinction must be made between the two conditions.

The patient struck down by myocardial infarction is usually aware that something unusual and grave has happened to him. Even when he has no pain he may feel ill in other ways. He is apprehensive and pale. He feels weak and sweats profusely, even though he is not excessively warm. He is frequently nauseated and may vomit. His pulse, although often normal, may be rapid and so faint as to be uncountable.

Because heart attacks are most dangerous in the first hour, there are a few facts that everyone should know; to be ignorant of these could result in the loss of a life, possibly your own. Sixty percent of the cases of myocardial infarction that end in death do so within one hour of onset; eighty-five percent of those who die do so within twenty-four hours. Seventy-seven percent of fatalities occur before the arrival of medical help. It is difficult to draw much consolation from these figures, but one conclusion is obvious: the sooner the victim of myocardial infarction receives professional assistance, the better his chances for survival.

Millions of dollars are being spent annually on the development and maintenance of coronary care units, which have significantly reduced mortality from myocardial infarction. Every discerning reader of forty or older should inquire whether there is a coronary care unit in his area and should make sure that no obstacles prevent his using it should he need its services.

The first few moments of the attack are critical. Muscle cells are being killed by a deficient supply of oxygen, and therefore the need for oxygen should be reduced to the lowest possible level. Walking requires more oxygen than standing, standing more than lying. The victim of myocardial infarction should be put at rest. It is safer to have him lie down on the street than to let him walk a block to a park bench. He should not try to drive home nor walk upstairs to his bedroom, because these efforts could result in the death of additional heart muscle and might mean the difference between recovery and fatality.

Whenever a heart attack is suspected, call for help. Don't delay. Do not waste time trying to make sure of the diagnosis; react as though it were a coronary and let the professionals decide whether you are right. I stress this because the greatest factor in fatal delay is indecision. Willingness to call for help early can mean the difference between life and death. Statistics from coronary care units suggest that the presumptive diagnosis of myocardial infarction is wrong in more than half the cases that reach the hospital. But if patients wait until diagnosis is assured, too many will have waited too long. Don't feel guilty about calling for help if you have even a suspicion that myocardial infarction has occurred.

Large amounts of oxygen continuously supplied to the heart muscle is the essential factor in preventing its death. Why, then, can't you supply pure oxygen from a tank kept for the purpose? You could, but it probably would do little good, because the oxygen available at the site of the injury is what counts; a blocked artery may prevent additional oxygen breathed from raising the oxygen level in the infarcted muscle. Nonetheless, oxygen is usually administered to ensure that the blood is as nourishing as possible.

Because the diagnosis of myocardial infarction and the care of the patient suffering its consequences must be handled by a physician and aides, this is not the place to give advice concerning those aspects of the disease. The victim may, however, feel less concerned if armed with a bit of knowledge about the tools available to the professionals who will be helping him. The most immediately available means of verifying a diagnosis of myocardial infarction is the electrocardiogram (EKG). The machine with which it is made, the electrocardiograph, can travel in the ambulance with a mobile unit; an electrocardiograph is usually found in every doctors' office and in the receiving room of every hospital. In most cases, the electrocardiogram will confirm or rule out a typical myocardial infarction, but a firm diagnosis awaits a more definitive investigation.

The family as well as the patient will be anxious to learn how gravely the heart has been damaged by the attack. There are tests to answer this question. The degenerating coronary muscle cells release a number of enzymes that can be detected in the blood stream and measured. The two most commonly tested for are known by their initials: LDH (lactic dehydrogenase) and CPK (creatinine phosphokinase). The amount of these substances in the blood in the first five days reflects the amount of heart tissue destroyed.

The patient and his family will also be eager to know how long the patient will be required to remain in the hospital and when it will be safe for him to go back to work. There are

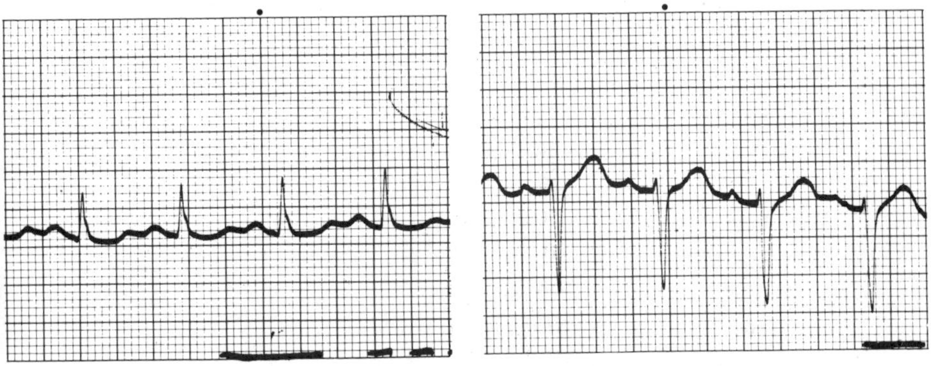

Electrocardiograms. The EKG shows if the rate and rhythm of the heartbeats are normal and if the contractions are weaker or stronger than normal. If a focal area of heart muscle is not performing properly, the shape and timing of the waves are altered in characteristic ways. By placing receptor discs at various points on the skin, a physician can measure currents passing through the heart muscle in twelve directions. Utilizing these leads, a physician can usually determine what part of the heart muscle is damaged. The EKG on the left is normal; the EKG on the right shows a myocardial infarction.

many qualifying conditions, but in an uncomplicated case the patient should expect to be hospitalized for an average of two weeks. Return to a light sedentary occupation such as desk work may be allowed in four more weeks. If he must perform physical labor, a longer period of rehabilitation may be required. Most recovered heart-attack patients are restricted to light or medium work; for example, lifting no more than fifty pounds.

The most important aspects of recovery from a myocardial infarction are complete rest for the first few days to reduce the load on the heart, quitting smoking (if the patient was a smoker), followed by diet, exercise, and, if indicated, medication. Any exertion whatsoever is ill advised until the danger of rupture of the heart wall has passed. If this is going to happen, it is apt to do so within the first ten days after the attack. Following this period, it becomes just as important to begin graduated exercise as it was to avoid it earlier. The heart is composed of muscle cells similar in many ways to the muscles of arms and legs. Muscle has to be exercised if it is to perform to its needed capabilities. The professional athlete knows the necessity of training seven days a week in order to remain in condition. The heart responds to exercise in the same way, but the exercise must be graduated to avoid serious damage from overload. Every physician will supply the postcoronary patient with an exercise schedule that must be rigidly observed.

What are the chances of recovery for the victim of myocardial infarction today? Again, there are many exceptions and conditions, but if we consider the vast majority of patients, those who reach professional help alive within an hour of onset have a survival rate very near 85 percent. Viewed in the light of the mortality statistics of years past, this is most reassuring. Knowledge and cooperation on the part of the public have played a significant role in the improvement of these figures.

6

Peripheral Vascular Disease

I have insisted that atherosclerosis of the coronary arteries is the most important disease of the cardiovascular system largely because of its frequency and the fact that life depends upon continuous performance by the heart. The coronary arteries are not the only ones affected by atherosclerosis, however; any medium-size or large artery can be. It is true that certain arteries are affected more often than others: the aorta, the coronaries, the carotid arteries (those to the brain), and those to the kidneys. Furthermore, certain regions of some arteries appear to be more vulnerable than others; among these are the first portion of the aorta as it emerges from the heart and the last portion as it divides in the lower abdomen to form the iliac arteries, which supply the legs. Atherosclerosis in the medium-size arteries located in tissues at some distance from the aorta is common enough to produce the diseases grouped under the heading peripheral vascular disease (PVD). The most important of these from the standpoint of incidence and mortality involves the arteries of the brain. I am referring to cerebral atherosclerosis, or stroke. Because hypertension plays such an important role in this disease, I shall consider the results of cerebral atherosclerosis in Chapter 8, after the discussion of high blood pressure.

Next in importance is the involvement of the arteries of the extremities in situations when the feet and hands do not receive an adequate supply of blood. Most of us have had transient episodes of "pins and needles," not necessarily caused by atherosclerosis. You should understand what is happening when they occur. Almost all peripheral vascular disease is caused by atherosclerosis and so it is appropriate to consider PVD as part of any discussion of atherosclerosis.

The formation of atheromatous plaques in the peripheral arteries is cumulative, just as it is in the coronary arteries. The symptoms come on gradually as the plaques slowly build up on the vessel walls and slowly narrow the arterial channel. When voluntary muscles are deprived of an adequate blood supply, they behave very much as the heart muscle does. For one thing, they become the site of transient pain. When this pain occurs in heart muscle it is called angina; when it occurs in peripheral muscle (the legs and, less often, the arms) it is called claudication.

Claudication is frequently described as a cramp, but intermittent claudication and true muscle cramp are not the same. The former is brought on by oxygen deprivation, the latter by abnormal nerve stimulation. We all have occasional muscle cramps. They come on while the muscle is at rest, often when you have been in bed for several hours. Claudication, on the other hand, manifests itself when the muscle is put to work and the demand for oxygen is increased. The pains usually last from one to two minutes. When the muscle is allowed to rest the pain ceases as suddenly as it appeared. The condition is encountered most frequently in the calf and ankle regions.

Intermittent claudication is the most common and most troublesome symptom of peripheral atherosclerosis. It increases progressively and eventually may prevent any exercise at all. In severe cases, the victim may be able to walk for only ten or fifteen minutes at a stretch before being obliged to rest. Symptoms are less severe when the extremity is positioned lower than the heart because the passage of blood is thereby facilitated by gravity.

There are symptoms other than pain. A "pins and needles" sensation (paresthesia) may occur and all feeling may give way to numbness. Because of poor circulation, the extremity may take on an unhealthy, flushed color. There may be loss of hair on the affected part and the skin may appear unnaturally smooth and shiny. (This is a sign of atrophy.) The nails of the fingers and toes, denied an adequate supply of fresh blood, become cracked and brittle. In advanced stages, constant pain may be experienced in the fingers or toes and ulceration of the skin and finally gangrene may follow.

Long before this catastrophe has befallen our hypothetical victim, he should have sought medical help. The condition of his peripheral arteries should have been evaluated by arteriography, a procedure in which a fluid that shows up on an x-ray is injected into the suspected vessel, which is then x-rayed in an attempt to find where the vessel channel has been narrowed. Sometimes a vessel transplant is possible. If the damage is not too extensive, the patient's atherosclerosis is evaluated and proper diet prescribed. Diabetes should always be suspected because it is known to contribute to the progress of atherosclerosis. Weight reduction and a weight reduction program are often beneficial, and the use of tobacco in any form will be forbidden. In extreme and advanced cases, amputation may be the only means of saving the patient's life from toxemia (blood poisoning). At the first definite indication of pain in the muscles of the extremities experienced during exercise, it is mandatory to seek professional help.

A less common but more serious complication of atherosclerosis occurs when the plaques build up in the aorta at the point where it divides to form the iliac arteries that supply blood to the legs. Although the mechanism is much the same as that of atherosclerosis when it occurs farther out in the vascular tree, the danger is that the blood is more apt to clot on the plaques at this site. A thrombus may eventually obstruct the outlets to both iliac arteries, cutting off the blood supply to the lower trunk and the legs and creating a surgical emergency.

The pain experienced as part of this blockage may occur in the legs, but it is more typically encountered in the lower back and buttocks. A common complaint among men is impotence caused by interference with the blood supply to the penis. High blood pressure is usually a part of the syndrome as well.

By the time the symptoms manifest themselves, it is usually

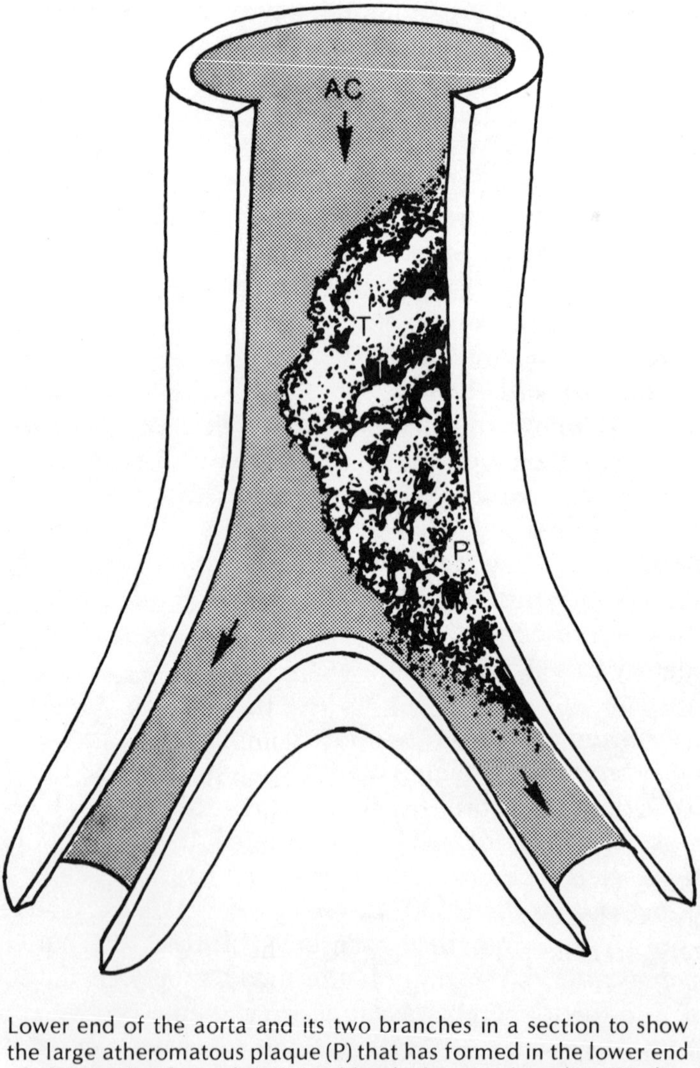

Lower end of the aorta and its two branches in a section to show the large atheromatous plaque (P) that has formed in the lower end of the aortic channel (AC). A blood clot, or thrombus (T), has formed on this plaque, partially closing the channels of both branches and so diminishing the flow of blood to the legs.

too late to correct the situation by means of conservative medical care and diet, but these measures should still be prescribed in an attempt to halt the atheromatous process. Surgical cure is possible; in most instances it is certainly worth a trial. If the aorta is not too badly destroyed it can sometimes be repaired. More often an arterial transplant or an artificial vessel (prosthesis) must be resorted to.

A third misfortune caused by atherosclerosis is the formation of aneurysms, blowouts of the arterial wall. Although aneurysms have been reported in the medium-size arteries of the extremities, they are much more common along the course of the aorta.

At one time not so many years ago, syphilitic infection was the leading cause of aneurysm. Now that the incidence of syphilis has been so dramatically lowered by the use of antibiotics, syphilitic aneurysm has become a rarity. Practically all aneurysms are now caused by atherosclerosis. There are two types.

The more common, the dissecting aneurysm, occurs most often in the abdominal aorta. An area of atheromatous destruction begins in the inner lining (intima) of the artery. It erodes into the aortic channel and forms an excavation into the middle, supportive layer (media). By the time atherosclerosis reaches this stage, it is usually accompanied by high blood pressure. The pressure of the blood within splits the eroded wall into layers and, if the outer wall holds, the splitting action extends by hydraulic pressure for a considerable distance along the course of the vessel.

This tearing of the wall into layers sometimes causes one of the most terrible pains imaginable. The lesion must be treated surgically, either by wrapping the vessel in plastic to support it or, if possible, by removing the damaged segment and replacing it with an artificial vessel segment.

The second type of aneurysm, saccular, is more apt to occur in the chest cavity. Like the dissecting aneurysm, it begins with an atheromatous lesion in the lining of the artery. The media is more extensively eroded and so weakened that its outer layers and the outer sheath of the aorta balloons outward and a saclike

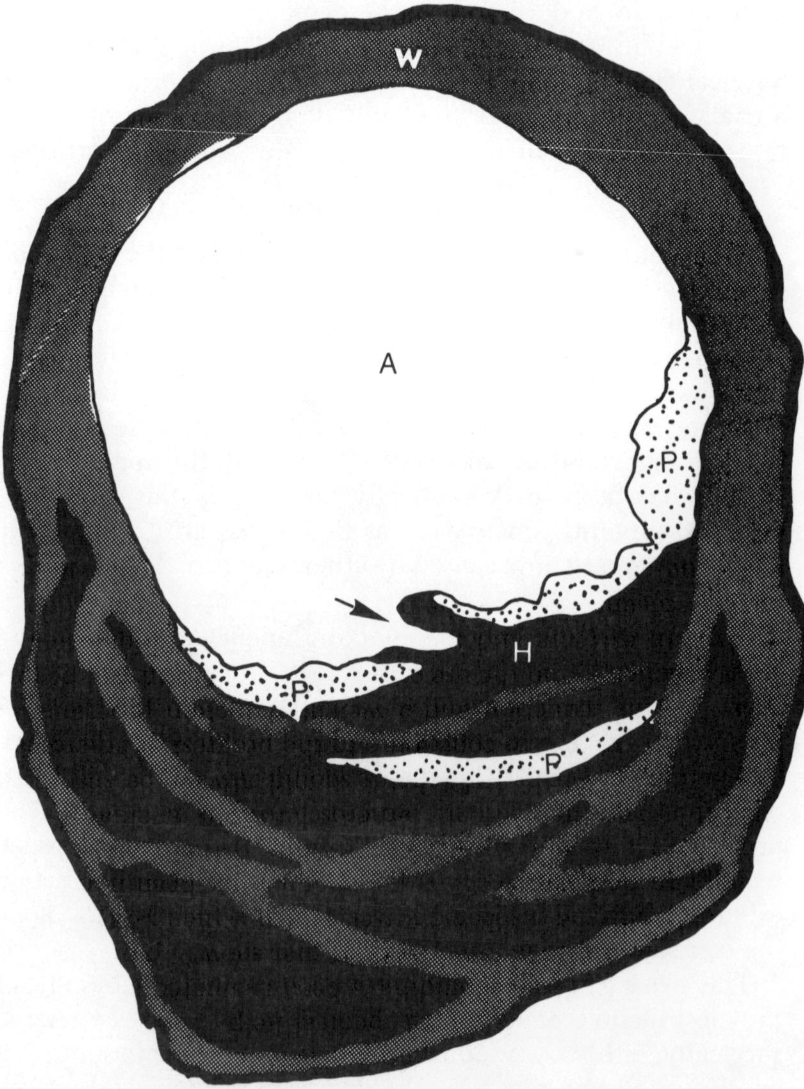

Dissecting aneurysm, seen in cross section through the abdominal portion of the aorta. (A) the aortic channel; (W) the normal aortic wall; (P) atheromatous plaques that have eroded into the channel at arrow, allowing outpouring blood to split the layers of the wall and form hematomas (H), masses of clotted blood, that have collected between the separated layers, thickening but weakening and distorting the vessel wall.

structure filled with blood forms. The saccular aneurysm may persist without symptoms for years, but more often it interferes with the function of a vital organ such as the heart or a lung. In the end, it is more apt to rupture, resulting in death by bleeding in a matter of minutes. This was the tragic finale of so many nineteenth-century romances, sure and deadly but mercifully swift. Now that the fury of syphilis has been contained and we are able to watch over the health of our aortas through

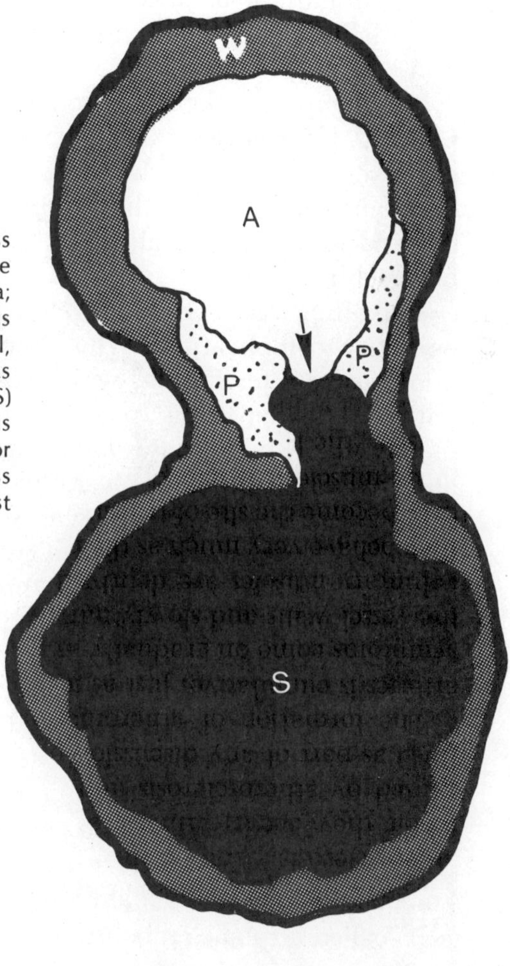

Saccular aneurysm, seen in cross section through the arch of the aorta. (W) the wall of the aorta; (A) its channel. An atheromatous plaque (P) has weakened the wall, allowing a blowout that has caused a saclike protrusion (S) filled with clotted blood. This sac may eventually rupture or the abdominal mass may press upon vital structures in the chest to cause pain.

the eyes of the x-ray and by supersonic scanning, a new breed of surgeons is treating our vessels surgically as our appendixes were once treated. Saccular aneurysms can and must be surgically repaired.

Perhaps the most dramatic of all vascular accidents is embolism. An embolus is any solid body carried in the blood stream. The most common solid body is a blood clot. When blood forms a clot on an arterial wall it is called a thrombus, but when it breaks loose and floats free it is called an embolus. When an embolus is carried to an artery whose channel is too small to allow it to pass—an inevitable eventuality—it plugs the smaller vessel. The whole process is called embolic occlusion.

The symptoms depend upon the particular artery that is plugged. If it is a very small artery in a tissue richly supplied by other vessels, there may be no symptoms at all. If the blockage occurs in a large artery that supplies a vital organ, death may be sudden. The latter, alas, is still frequent, though it used to be much more so.

Embolism was once the surgeon's bête noire, a frequent postoperative complication. What happened was that an operation, usually for hernia, was successfully completed and the patient returned to his room in good condition. Because any movement would cause pain and inconvenience, he was allowed to lie quietly for several days. This inactivity, together with other factors associated with surgical manipulation, often caused a thrombus to form in a peripheral vein. Then, when the patient finally did move, the thrombus broke loose and was carried to the heart by the venous blood. It passed through the heart and out into the pulmonary artery to the lungs. There, when it reached a smaller branch, it was stopped. The patient often died within moments. The shock engendered by the report of this event was almost as traumatic to the surgeon as it was to the patient's family. You may have wondered why modern hospital attendants are so eager to get patients up and active as soon as possible after an operation. Avoiding pulmonary embolism is one of the main reasons.

So-called airplane embolism is important enough to warrant

a note of caution here. When you spend several hours in a single position that puts pressure on a large venous channel, the return flow of blood may be slowed sufficiently to precipitate intravenous clotting. Anyone packed tightly in a crowded airplane, the edge of the seat pressing on the underside of the knees over the course of a long flight, is subject to these conditions. When he rises and straightens his legs, the thrombus that may have formed is loosened to become an embolus. Solution: on long flights, be sure to walk the aisles at intervals.

All of the above vascular diseases, with the exception of embolism, are caused by atherosclerosis. Atheromatous deterioration of the arterial wall is the villain of the piece, although the layperson rarely sees that name on the playbill. By the time symptoms occur it is usually too late to do much about the disease by conservative medical means. The innocent but uninformed patient is obliged to accept help through surgery. The time is long overdue for atherosclerosis to be treated before it begins. Certain components of our diets should be recognized for what they are: insidious and malicious killers. If our children never acquire a taste for them, they will never miss them.

To see the complications of atherosclerosis in their proper perspective, we should briefly consider certain other diseases that affect our blood vessels. Perhaps the most interesting group and surely the one the public understands least are those conditions brought on by allergy. We began to learn the truth about allergies during the late 1940s and 1950s. We erroneously called them the collagen diseases because our attention was misdirected by microscopic changes observed in the vessel walls, which some pathologists interpreted improperly. The diseases included in this group are lupus erythematosus, its cousin polyarteritis, and possibly scleroderma and dermatomyositis. Also included by some is a much more common disease, rheumatoid arthritis. Had we been a bit brighter back in the 1950s we would have recognized that we already had a working laboratory model for the study of these conditions in serum sickness.

The principles of allergy are now well known. The cells of our body are made up largely of proteins, thousands of combinations of amino acids, each combination with its individual hallmark. Our cells do not take kindly to foreigners. When a protein with an unknown hallmark (an antigen) is introduced into our tissues, it is greeted with animosity. Certain cells copy the antigen and take it back to lymph nodes and spleen. There, specific cells are produced and sent out to deal with the matter. This causes inflammation which is called the antigen-antibody reaction. In the turmoil of this chemical battle, the supportive tissue (collagen) of the vessel wall is injured.

A portion of the wall of very small arteries is affected because the antigen (whose identity is usually unknown) and the antibody formed to deal with it are chemical substances transported in the blood stream. The channels of the minute vessels are their battleground. The injured area swells and closes the vessel passage. The blood that is obstructed clots. A microscopic area of allergic inflammation occurs. Millions of these areas affecting different tissue regions constitute the various diseases of this group, the nature of the disease depending upon the tissue predominantly involved.

Lupus (properly systemic lupus erythematosus or SLE) is one of these. It affects women about nine times more frequently than it does men. It usually begins during adolescence or in the early twenties, but it can start as late as age fifty. The most common complaint is pain in the joints. This symptom usually leads to a mistaken diagnosis of rheumatoid arthritis. When the skin is involved, as it is in nearly half the cases, the diagnosis becomes obvious. A clearly demarcated area of skin rash occurs on the cheeks and across the bridge of the nose in the shape of a butterfly. (Indeed, it is called a butterfly rash.) Fever and a feeling of profound weakness are usually experienced. The disease most commonly occurs in episodes that last several weeks, with intervals during which the patient is quite free of symptoms. Exposure to sunlight may precipitate an episode. In time, the arterioles of the kidneys are involved; then the patient has and often dies of nephritis. The average life expectancy after the disease is well established is about five years, but some sufferers have lived much longer.

Polyarteritis nodosa affects men about three times more often than it does women, and usually in a somewhat older age group. Although the arterioles may be involved as they are in lupus, the brunt of the damage is borne by somewhat larger arterial channels. The type of destruction in the wall of the vessel is quite similar to that of lupus but the lesion is larger, forming a node of inflammatory reaction.

The patient is apt to suffer fever and weakness, loss of weight, and pains in the joints and muscles. Because the small arteries within the abdomen are often involved, the symptoms are related to the gastrointestinal tract—nausea, vomiting, abdominal pain, and diarrhea. When one or more of these symptoms occurs and none of the other systems appear to be involved, a mistaken diagnosis of acute abdominal crisis may be made and the patient subjected to an unneeded abdominal operation. As in lupus, the kidneys are eventually affected in more than half the cases, and then hypertension is added to the patient's woes.

Scleroderma and dermatomyositis are diseases with many features similar to those of lupus and polyarteritis. Their causes are less clearly understood than those of lupus and polyarteritis, but they probably belong to the same disease group. In scleroderma, most of the lesions are in the skin; in dermatomyositis they are chiefly in the muscles. Their symptoms are related to the areas of maximum involvement.

Finally, two vascular diseases should be mentioned for the sake of completeness. They are Raynaud's disease and Buerger's disease.

Raynaud's disease, technically acrocyanosis, is a curious phenomenon in which apparently transitory contraction spasms occur in the arteries that supply the fingers and toes. These extremities usually turn dead white at first and then become cyanotic (blue). The color changes may be accompanied by stiffness and numbness. The oxygen deprivation is not so severe as to cause tissue destruction, so ulceration and gangrene are not part of the disease. The cause of this condition is unknown, but attacks are usually brought on by exposure to cold.

Buerger's disease, or thromboangiitis obliterans, is much more serious. This condition is almost always associated with atherosclerosis. In fact, some people prefer to think of it not as a specific entity but as an expression of severe atherosclerosis predominantly involving the arteries of the extremities. There are several features of the disease that argue against this belief: the involvement of veins and nerves as well as arteries, and its persistent relation to the use of tobacco.

This disease attacks young males, almost all of whom smoke in excess. The earliest manifestations are usually seen in the fingers and toes, where the small arteries are affected. The fingers and toes turn white, then blue, and finally red. This patriotic display is accompanied by pain and the appearance in the skin of small nodules that are red and tender. Pains commonly occur in the feet. In this disease, too, there is sensitivity to cold. The oxygen deprivation in these cases usually progresses to tissue destruction. Ulcers eventually appear, usually on the tips of the fingers. After these, gangrene can be expected unless the progress of the disease is halted. The fingers and toes turn black and must be amputated. Unfortunately, however, amputation does nothing to stop the disease. Next the hands and feet are affected and they, too, may have to be sacrificed. The arterial changes may progress to involve all of both extremities. I once encountered a case in a man in his thirties who had to have both arms and both legs amputated.

Little is known about the cause of Buerger's disease, but tobacco seems to be implicated in some way. Some patients who have scrupulously avoided use of all forms of the plant have enjoyed complete recovery; others have not. An inexplicable phenomenon is the stubborn persistence with which some patients, knowing the facts, continue to smoke, even after amputations have been necessary.

Atherosclerosis affects any and all of the medium-size and large arteries of the body. When it affects those of the heart it produces heart attack. When it affects those of the brain it may result in stroke. When the vessels of the extremities are involved, the blood supply is depleted and the symptoms of peripheral vascular disease result. Although the cause is the same, the manifestations of these three conditions are quite different. The layperson frequently does not realize that the preventive treatment for the three most common serious diseases of mankind is avoiding atherosclerosis.

Another complication of atherosclerosis is hypertension, or high blood pressure. This condition is considered in the following chapter.

7

Hypertension

Hypertension (high blood pressure) is an extremely complicated disease. For the sake of simplicity, cases are usually divided into two types: essential (or simple) and secondary hypertension. Secondary hypertension means that the blood-pressure elevation is the result of a known cause. Those cases in which the cause is not identifiable are called essential or simple hypertension. Both types must be treated, and the treatment varies with the cause. In essential hypertension, cooperation between patient and physician is especially important because diet, exercise, and weight control are central features of the therapy. There are many causes of secondary hypertension, some of them so complicated that many physicians have only the vaguest concept of the underlying mechanism. What chance, then, has a layperson of understanding the most common disease of industrialized peoples?

It is generally estimated that 20 percent of Americans over the age of thirty-five have high blood pressure. Essential hypertension almost always begins between the ages of thirty-five and fifty. In the great majority of cases it is controllable by medication and diet. In only a small percentage of cases will the condition eventually cause death, and then not until it has persisted for close to twenty years. In those over sixty, however, hypertension is, along with atherosclerosis, the most common cause of cerebrovascular accident (stroke), which is second only to heart attack as the most common cause of death due to cardiovascular disease.

About 5 percent of all cases of hypertension, whether essential or secondary, either begin as or become malignant hypertension. Unless vigorously treated, this most severe type of high blood pressure progresses fairly steadily to cause death by kidney failure among its younger victims and stroke in its older ones in a matter of months.

The most important things for the layperson to know about hypertension are that it is exceedingly common, that the great majority of cases can be alleviated by simple treatment, and that failure to recognize and deal with early hypertension may result in stroke or heart attack later on. After age thirty everyone should have his or her blood pressure taken every two or three years; after forty it should be done every year; and after sixty-five, every six months.

Before going any further, let us be certain that everyone understands what hypertension is. When the heart muscle contracts, it forces blood into the arteries. At that moment the pressure in the arteries is at its maximum. The contracted state of the heart muscle is called systole; diastole is the name for the relaxed state. Systolic pressure is the maximum pressure recorded during contraction of the heart muscle. When the heart muscle relaxes, the valves between the heart and the arteries close behind the blood, which is then additionally propelled forward by contraction waves in the arteries. As the blood disperses into the arterial branches, the pressure falls. The lowest level of pressure is achieved at the moment before the heart contracts again; this is called the diastolic pressure. The contraction and relaxation cycle occurs with each heartbeat. Systolic pressure depends on a number of factors, such as the pulse rate and the force of contraction; diastolic pressure is unaffected by these mitigating factors. Because it does not vary from moment to moment, diastolic pressure is the more dependable. Nonetheless, both figures are significant and are always stated together, systolic pressure first, then diastolic. For example, "120 over 80" represents a systolic pressure of 120 and a diastolic pressure of 80.

Let us use a greatly simplified analogy to examine the factors that maintain blood pressure. Keep in mind, however, that the reality is considerably more complicated. Imagine a closed fluid-conduction system consisting of a pump and a circuit of elastic tubing that leads the fluid away from the pump into a tank and from the tank back into the pump. Fluid may be drained from the tank and extra fluid may be added to it. Now we start the pump. The amount of pressure in the system will depend upon the force of the pump, the output of each pump stroke, and the volume of the fluid returned to the pump. It will also depend upon the capacity of the tubes. These are only a few of the important factors that apply to the body, and each

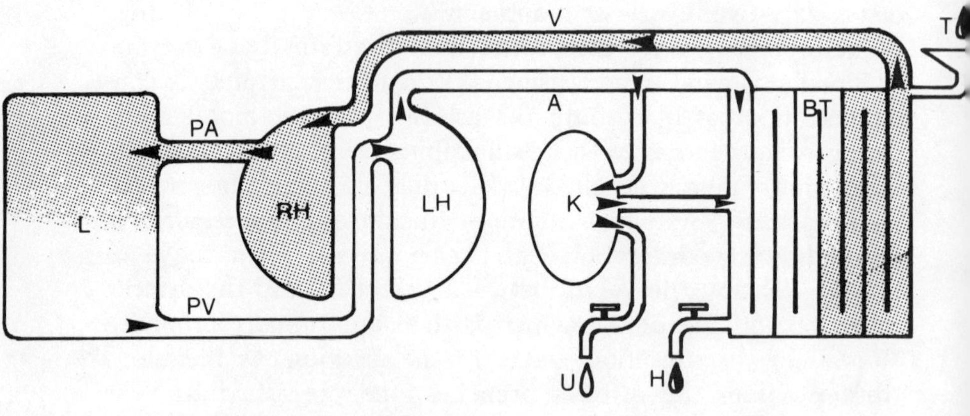

Schematic diagram of the cardiovascular system. Pump (LH), representing the left heart, propels blood through the arteries (A) into tank (BT), representing the body tissues. Its oxygen taken by body cells, the blood flows via the veins (V) into the right heart (RH). From here it is sent through the pulmonary artery (PA) to tank (L), representing the lungs, where it is reoxygenated and returned to the left heart through the pulmonary vein (PV). Arterial blood also goes to the kidneys (K), where it is cleansed of its wastes. The clean blood is returned to (BT). The wastes and excess fluids escape in the urine (U). Thus there are two systems with differing pressures: the arterial and the venous. When the pressure in one system changes the other must eventually change, too.

factor is affected in turn by a number of mechanisms, some of which are still not understood.

To continue our analogy, under ordinary circumstances the pressure is greatest as the fluid leaves the pump. This is analogous to systolic pressure. The elastic tubes first dilate, then squeeze the fluid along its course into the tank. Suppose we open a small valve on the tank; this is analogous to a hemorrhage. If enough fluid is lost, the amount in the system becomes inadequate to refill the pump (heart). In the human body, this would induce shock; the heart would pump faster to compensate for the reduced output of blood. This would manifest itself in a rapid pulse and a dramatic drop in pressure, resulting in fainting. Now suppose that we add fluid to the tank, raising the level above normal. Fluid takes up space, thereby increasing the pressure in the system. We could obtain the same result of elevated pressure by causing the elastic tubes to contract, thus reducing the capacity of the circulatory system.

Blood pressure is expressed as the number of millimeters of a column of mercury which corresponds to the amount of pressure necessary to compress an artery. The test is a familiar one to all, but how many of us know what the doctor is doing when he wraps that tourniquet around our arm? The tourniquet consists of a rubber balloon wrapped in a cloth bag; it may be used on any extremity, the arm being the most common. Pressure within the balloon is increased when air is pumped into it. When an artery is compressed, the blood flowing past the compression makes a distinctive sound that can be recognized by the physician with the aid of a stethoscope. When the blood flow is completely stopped there is no sound, as is the case when the flow is completely unobstructed.

The physician pumps air into the balloon until the flow through the arteries is stopped. He then gradually decreases the pressure of the tourniquet until he begins to hear the blood flow. He notes that point on the scale of the sphygmomanometer, the measuring device attached to the tourniquet. He has thus recorded the systolic pressure, the peak pressure within the artery under his stethoscope. Next he releases more air from the balloon, further reducing the pressure on the artery. When the blood passing through the artery is no longer obstructed, the sound he heard through his stethoscope fades and disappears. The number of millimeters registered on the sphygmomanometer at that point is equivalent to the diastolic pressure.

Blood pressure readings are not immutable figures. An individual's pressure varies a few points from hour to hour, depending upon the kind of exercise taken, the position of the body—standing, sitting, or lying—and the emotional state. In fact, minute blood-pressure alterations are used in lie-detector tests to infer the subject's emotional reactions to various questions.

It would be misleading to state a figure and insist that all those with blood pressures above it have hypertension. We need some guideposts, so we set limits of "normal" blood pressure and adjust them to fit individual cases. Women tolerate high pressures better than men do, for reasons that are not understood. Recent studies suggest that persistent blood pressures above 150/95 require treatment, especially in young males.

To review, blood pressure depends on the amount of blood in the circulatory system and the pressure exerted upon it by the pumping of the heart and the squeezing action of the elastic-walled arteries which carry it. When one or both of these factors is increased, or if the capacity of the system as a whole is decreased, hypertension results. Any discussion of causes must therefore take each factor into account.

An increase in blood volume and a contraction of the volume of the vascular system are the two most common alterations that occur. Many factors influence these changes; I shall cite only a few of the simpler ones in the hope that they will help you comprehend the complex problems of hypertension.

One of the most significant influences on the amount of circulating blood is the electrolyte balance. The body uses a number of minerals (electrolytes) in its routine metabolism. Since they are essential to health, several checks and balances are required to keep their levels in the tissues and blood constant. For example, one of these minerals, calcium, is essential to the transport of impulses along the nerve fibers. It combines with phosphorous to form a crystalline salt that provides rigidity to bones and teeth. Phosphorous is also necessary in the metabolism of protein, which allows us to build new cells for growth and tissue maintenance. Sodium is essential to the maintenance of fluid balance. It resides in free body fluids, lymph, and blood plasma. Its analog, potassium, is found within the cells. When the sodium level rises, the potassium level falls, and vice versa. Each is important in maintaining osmotic pressure.

When the sodium concentration in the blood is increased, fluid is withdrawn from elsewhere in the body to restore the level to normal; if there is more sodium, there must be more fluid to maintain the balance. The first place from which fluid is drawn is the intestinal tract, which has the effect of causing thirst. Next, the lymph that bathes cells gives up fluid, causing dehydration. Finally, fluid is drawn from the cells themselves. Cells do not tolerate fluid loss because water is a necessary component in their metabolic routine. The fluid drawn from these sources is brought into and held in the blood stream, adding to its volume, which, depending on the capacity of the vascular system, may increase blood pressure.

Among their many functions, the kidneys regulate the excretion and retention of sodium. Each kidney is made up of over a million units called nephrons, tiny threadlike structures consisting of a tubule (small tube) with a bulblike clump of capillaries (the smallest blood vessels) at one end called the glomerulus. The glomerulus acts as a mechanical strainer, holding back blood cells, sugar, and protein while allowing water, sodium, potassium, and body wastes to pass. The tubules must salvage any important blood constituents that the glomeruli have allowed to pass through and return them to the blood stream.

The way in which the sodium level is regulated is complex. When blood pressure falls to a level that prevents nutrients and oxygen from being delivered in adequate amounts to the various cells throughout the body, a message is sent to certain cells within the kidneys, which step up their production of a chemical substance called renin. Released into the blood, renin finds angiotensinogin, a chemical substance formed in the liver. These two combine to form a third substance, angiotensin, which has two important functions in the body. It stimulates the adrenal glands to secrete aldosterone, which in turn causes the nephron tubules to excrete more potassium and retain sodium. It also causes the blood vessels to contract, thus reducing the capacity of the arterial system. This is the classical manner in which nature works: trial and error, until after thousands of years of failure she gets it right.

Sodium retention is a significant factor in hypertension because the greater the concentration of sodium in the blood, the more fluid is brought in from other body sources to balance it; this increases blood volume. We obtain most of our sodium in the form of ordinary table salt, sodium chloride. The layperson has been told that salt causes high blood pressure and should, therefore, be avoided. This caveat is not necessarily so for everyone. Salt does not cause hypertension; the *retention* of salt leads to the disease, and the cause of retention can be, among other things, a malfunctioning kidney.

While most of us eat more salt than we should, people with an inherited tendency toward hypertension should be particularly wary because their kidneys, for reasons that are still unclear, are set to retain abnormal quantities of sodium. Salt is a valuable flavor adjunct; it should be used intelligently. It should certainly not be abused, but I see no reason to needlessly restrict it. As is so often the case, moderation seems the best path. It is best not to fall into the habit of using a great deal of salt, even though it may not be harmful to you at this particular point in your life. Most people find that with free usage they tend to increase the amount of salt they add to their food to the point that considerably more than moderate amounts are used. Too many people salt before tasting rather than the reverse, which is what we should do. Salt substitutes are a help, but they do not taste much like salt. Commercial table salt that is half sodium chloride and half potassium chloride substantially reduces sodium intake, but getting used to less salty tastes seems the wiser approach.

There are many reasons why the kidneys produce abnormal amounts of renin. Let us look at some of the more important ones. The most essential function of the kidneys is to filter wastes from the blood. How well they do that depends on how much blood passes through them in a given period of time. We should not be surprised that nature has provided a number of safeguards to ensure adequate blood passage. One of these is the secretion of renin. This check-and-balance rationale hinges on the assumption that the higher the blood pressure, the greater the amount of blood forced through the kidneys. Unfortunately, it does not always work that way.

If sodium retention is the most common cause of hypertension (through increased blood volume), the second most common is reduction in the capacity of the arterial system as a result of several influences. Contraction of the arterial walls reduces the diameter of their channels and thus reduces their capacity. This occurs as the result of a complicated chain of chemical reactions that, as we have seen, starts in the kidneys. Reduction in the kidneys' blood supply because of a reduction in the diameter of the channels of the vessels that carry blood to them can result from atherosclerosis. This type of arterial disease affects, among others, the arteries that serve the kidneys. Because atherosclerosis is a cumulative disease and affects the renal arteries in the latter half of life, it may not be severe enough to be a factor in elevating blood pressure.

A second type of vessel sclerosis, called arteriolarsclerosis, is much less common than atherosclerosis, but in older people it frequently affects the renal vessels severely enough to restrict the blood supply to the kidneys.

Whereas the large and medium-size arteries are affected in atherosclerosis, only the smallest, the arterioles, are affected in arteriolarsclerosis. Their walls are greatly thickened at the expense of the diameter of their channels. The capacity of the circulatory system is greatly reduced; consequently the pressure of the blood must rise, and the result is hypertension. We are not sure whether the thickening of the walls of the arterioles causes hypertension or whether essential hypertension demands stronger vessels and so thickens the walls. All that we know is that there is a concomitant rise in blood pressure and a thickening of small arterial walls, and that in the earliest stages the mechanism is probably unrelated to sodium retention.

The organs most prominently affected by arteriolarsclerosis are the kidneys. An arteriole supplies each clump of capillary

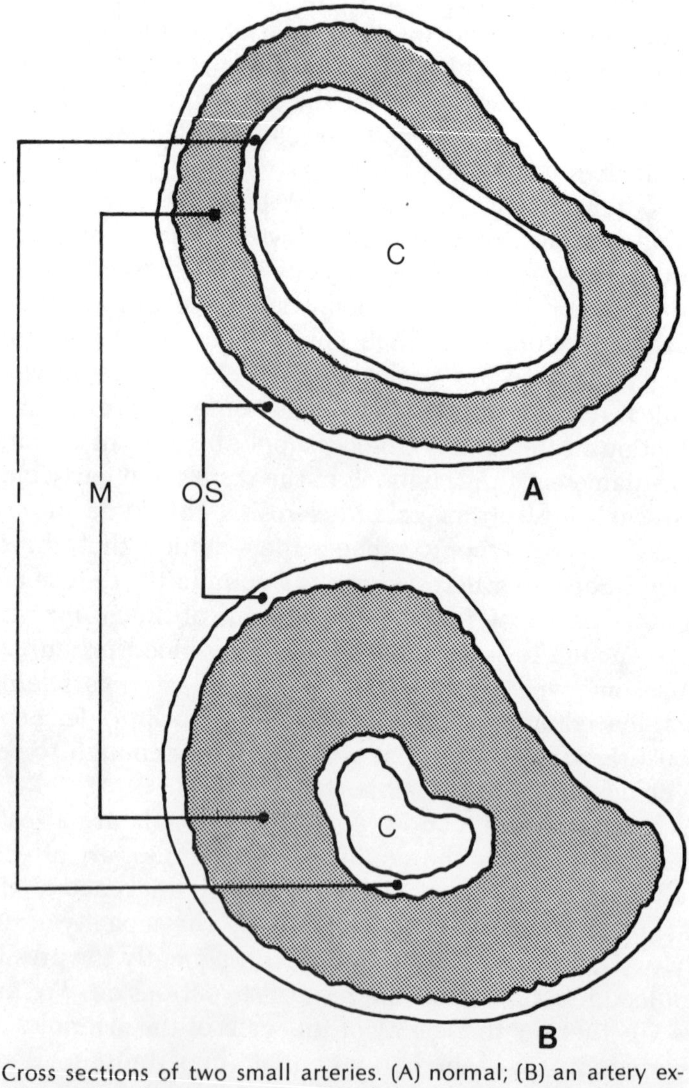

Cross sections of two small arteries. (A) normal; (B) an artery exhibiting the changes of arteriolarsclerosis. In this type of arteriosclerosis the middle arterial coat (M) is greatly thickened at the expense of the channel (C); the inner arterial sheath (I) and the outer sheath (OS) are not greatly changed. This type of vascular sclerosis is different from atherosclerosis, in which cholesterol plaques form in the inner sheath. Because only large and medium-size arteries are involved in atherosclerosis, the vascular bed is not greatly diminished.

vessels that make up the nephron. The narrowed arteriolar channel reduces the blood flow through the kidneys, the renin-secreting cells go to work, and the end result is an increase in angiotensin, which stimulates the manufacture of aldosterone, causing an eventual conservation of sodium. In addition to triggering the secretion of aldosterone, angiotensin also causes the muscles of the walls of the arterioles to contract, resulting in a rise in blood pressure. Thus two distinct mechanisms are caused by the same hormone: retention of sodium and reduction in the capacity of the circulatory system because of contraction of arteriolar walls. The two work to attain the same objective: the elevation of blood pressure.

When pressures are persistently elevated to or above 160/95 in males or 160/100 in females, it is called hypertension. Pressures of this dimension are usually without symptoms, but not without damaging effects, which explains why we should all have our pressure taken periodically as a matter of routine. When the hypertensive level is reached, therapy should be contemplated to keep the pressure from going into an even higher stage, one that may be less amenable to treatment.

Because hypertension is so common, it has created a considerable interest among the public along with a considerable body of myth concerning its cause and treatment. It was once believed that people of certain emotional and body types were more vulnerable to certain diseases, including hypertension. Under this theory, if a person were known to have a violent temper, particularly if he were prone to public tantrums, he was supposed to be a likely candidate for high blood pressure. Cadaverous types, prone to worry about inconsequentials, or those forced to labor under severe and continued mental stress, were also supposed to be vulnerable. I know of no valid statistical proof for these assertions. Nor do I know of any physical or emotional situations that can be shown unequivocally to cause sustained hypertension, although bouts of emotional stress may cause temporary elevations in blood pressure. There is a racial and genetic predisposition to the disease. However, this cannot be interpreted to mean that body type and emotional state are causally related to hypertension.

Recently we have been hearing a good deal about biofeedback (a bad and inaccurate term) as a method for treating hypertension. It is true that temporary reductions of blood pressure are sometimes attained by this practice, but never, to my knowledge, in severe hypertensives. There is no reason to believe that the method is practical, curative, or usable by any but a few suggestible subjects. Hypertension should be treated by standard remedies administered by experienced medical personnel. A hypertensive solely in the hands of a biofeedback enthusiast may be sacrificing a chance for a cure.

Although the customary treatment for hypertension is usually simple and relatively inexpensive, it should never be undertaken without professional guidance. The overweight patients will probably be asked to reduce. They will probably be advised to avoid salt, because by this time their kidneys are probably retaining more sodium than they should. A mild diuretic—a drug that removes sodium, potassium, and water through the kidneys in the form of urine—may be prescribed. In nine out of ten cases such measures will suffice. But if a diastolic pressure of well over 100 has been sustained for a considerable length of time, reduction in pressure may be much more difficult to achieve.

Statistics based on large numbers of people with simple hypertension indicate a life expectancy without treatment of about twenty years from the time the first abnormal pressure is recorded. With proper treatment, life expectancy is restored almost to normal.

The earliest symptom noticed by the hypertensive is usually a headache. Because headaches are so common, caused as they are by everything from eye strain to the intemperate use of alcohol the previous night, most people take aspirin and ignore it. When it persists or recurs, they may put it down to an attack of sinusitis. It may be weeks before this symptom suggests a visit to a physician, who might suspect the presence of high blood pressure. Hypertensive headache usually occurs in the morning on awakening and passes away spontaneously in two or three hours. It is characteristically located at the back of the head. It may be accompanied by dizziness and a tired feeling. When the hypertension is well established, the sufferer is often aware that his heart is beating more rapidly and forcefully than normal; we call this palpitations. If left untreated, nosebleed, blurring of vision, and finally shortness of breath and chest pain (angina) eventually develop, because the heart becomes exhausted from working against the increased pressure. At this stage, various organs are suffering from inadequate blood supplies. If the disease is permitted to progress without treatment, death can be expected. In those between thirty-five and fifty years of age, the kidneys usually go first, and death from uremia is the result; in older people, stroke brought on by hypertension will be the cause of death.

In about 5 percent of all cases of high blood pressure, particularly in the age group between thirty-five and forty-five, the changes in the arterioles seem to get out of hand. This type of high blood pressure is called malignant essential hypertension. It is the most dreaded of the hypertensive diseases because it strikes in early middle age and is rapidly fatal. The changes in the arterioles are much more prominent than in other types of hypertension. The blood pressure soars to 240/140 and higher. The diagnosis is usually easy to make by a simple eye examination using an ophthalmoscope; this is a routine part of a physical examination. The area where the optic nerve enters the retina will appear swollen and gray. Visual changes are more pronounced and sometimes progress to blindness. The headache is very severe, often accompanied by vomiting. The brain swells, which can lead to transient attacks of paralysis. Eventually there are convulsions, stupor, and coma. Death usually occurs from kidney failure in about two years. Even with adequate treatment, only about a third of those afflicted live five years. For a reason that has never been adequately explained, malignant essential hypertension is much more common among blacks than whites.

There are several important things you should know about hypertension. First, you should have your pressure taken sometime in early life, perhaps around the age of twenty. If it is normal, you need not be concerned until around thirty, when you should have it tested every two or three years; after forty, it should be measured once a year; and after sixty-five, once every six months. If you are reading this too late to start from step one, pick up at the appropriate age. Your retinal vessels should be examined through an ophthalmoscope during every physical examination, because the retina is the only place where the arterioles can be observed adequately. When typical changes occur in the retinal tissues, they are highly significant in arteriolarsclerosis; observable changes may not occur in these vessels in atherosclerosis. If at any time your diastolic pressure is consistently recorded above ninety-five, a few chemical tests will be ordered. Only rarely will hospitalization be required for more extensive tests. The aim is to be sure that the hypertension does not have an underlying, or secondary, cause, such as congenital malformation of the kidney or aorta or, in females, a side effect of oral contraceptives. If secondary hypertension is ruled out, the therapeutic regimen already described will be undertaken.

Keep in mind that hypertension provokes and hastens atherosclerosis, especially in those who are over fifty. An elevation of pressure within the arteries apparently damages their walls and causes their supportive tissue to increase in bulk. This damage is followed by scar formation and thickening of the walls, which in turn reduces the capacity of the arterial system. The combination of these two conditions, the weakening of the vessel wall (atherosclerosis) and the increase in pressure within (hypertension), results in stroke, the most common cause of death in elderly peoples of industrialized populations.

8

Cerebrovascular Disease

"The difference in mind between man and the higher animals, great as it is, certainly is one of degree and not of kind." So said Charles Darwin almost a century ago. This assertion made more attractive a new kind of investigation, one unhampered by secular or religious bias. Carl Sagan wrote, in *The Dragons of Eden*, "Workings [of the brain] are a consequence of anatomy, physiology and nothing more." E. O. Wilson, in his important and admirable book, *On Human Nature*, said it more succinctly and poetically: "We are biological and our souls cannot fly free."

Those of us accustomed to reading accounts of quantum mechanics, space exploration, particle physics, and the coding on the hereditary helix accept this fact as a matter of course. There are, however, many prominent sectarians and even a few scientists in the modern world who hold sociobiology to be a denigration of mankind. For the purposes of our discussion we shall profit by a little knowledge of brain anatomy and its derivations, but we need not become enmeshed in the polemics concerning its higher functions. We can afford to leave that in the hands of psychologists, philosophers, and metaphysicians—and may God help them!

Perhaps the greatest obstacle in the search to understand brain function is the lack of a control implement with which to carry out the research. It is a fundamental truth that brain activity has to be measured by brain activity.

One of the modes of the study of the mind has been provided by the study of brains with focal areas of damage caused by deprivation of blood supply. When any tissue is so deprived the area is said to be ischemic. When a record was made of the changes in mental activity of patients who had suffered damage to the blood supply of their brains, and then a study was done of the anatomy of the ischemic organ, a great deal was learned about normal brain function.

When damage to the brain occurs because of interference in its blood supply, we call it cerebrovascular accident or, more commonly, stroke. Every intelligent person should understand something of the nature of cerebrovascular accidents, why they occur, how they may affect life, and what can be done to avoid them.

But first a word about the anatomy and the derivations of the human brain. In terms of the history of our world, our brains are not very old; indeed, they are very young. If we imagine the entire existence of the universe in terms of one calendar year, the evolution of man and his brain would require less than the last hour of the last day. When we consider the evolution of the human brain, we see that the last stage is a recapitulation of the whole. In man's hindbrain we see the beginning, that with which the fish and his brethren must be content. A bit further up is the midbrain, which suffices for the reptiles; and finally the elaborately folded forebrain, which includes the complex cerebral cortex. In the case of our central nervous system, evolution came about largely by addition; little was discarded on the long journey upward. By studying the brains of the lower forms we are able to extrapolate data that otherwise would be impossible to appreciate.

The brain maintains a state of awareness through a flood of incoming sensations that begin in our sense organs—eyes, nose, ears, tongue, skin. These receptors—the optic (sight), olfactory (smell), auditory (hearing), gustatory (taste), tactile (feeling), and kinesthetic (position)—have been specifically modified to appreciate the signals that reach them from the environment. They initiate and send impulses, minute bursts of electrical energy, up the nerves to the spinal cord and brain in the form of a code, just as electrical impulses are sent along a wire, to a machine which can decode the message into a telegram. In the central nervous system, these code signals are integrated with millions of other signals continuously pouring in. Experience conditions the pathways so that eventually the impulses are guided through complex integration patterns, thus producing the images that we interpret as the world around us.

Should something go wrong with the production of these impulses in the sensory organ, with their passage along the nerve, or with their integration once they have reached the brain, the image may appear distorted. If someone's actions appear a bit queer it is probably because some alteration has occurred in the mechanics of impulse processing. Visions, auditory hallucinations, and strange conclusions are no more mystical than the pain that occurs in the gall bladder when a stone upsets its normal function by blocking a duct. When trouble develops in the brain's blood supply, ischemic lesions occur that alter brain function. We may encounter amnesia (impaired memory), dysgraphia (impaired writing), ataxia (failure of muscle coordination), dysarthria (impaired speaking), and dozens of other coordination impairments and behavior alterations. The recognition and location of these alterations and their causes constitute the discipline of neurology.

We need only consider the major vascular lesions that are extremely common. But a word about impulse pathways before we describe the lesions that disrupt them. When an impulse that originated in a sensory organ reaches the central nervous system, it is cataloged by the complicated system of synapses (organic transistors) and sent on to the higher coordinating network of cells. This constitutes recent memory. If the impulses are repeated sufficiently, the organic transistor gates are conditioned so that the pathways become semipermanent. This is long-term memory or learning.

If, on its arrival at the first set of synapses in the spinal cord, the impulse is coordinated with other impulses reaching this site, it may be sent out to its objective in the peripheral tissues without ever reaching the brain and without becoming conscious. This is called a reflex. Much of the knowledge that we inherit is reflexive in nature. Early in this century, Ivan Pavlov showed that with experience many reflexes may be conditioned. More recent work makes it appear that pathways in the higher centers can also be conditioned so that the autonomic nervous system can be controlled to a degree. When this is accomplished the person undergoing the training may be able to use concentration to control his sense of pain, his pulse rate, and to a degree, his blood pressure (although not in cases of established hypertension). This type of concentration has been called meditation, and a good deal of meaningless claptrap has been added to heighten its mystical aspects. Sensations may be distorted to produce visual images and auditory hallucinations. The Orient discovered this phenomenon centuries ago. Failing to understand its physiological explanation, Eastern mystics worked it into a number of quasi-religious philosophies. Modern psychologists are only now beginning to understand the mechanics of these strange goings-on.

When the impulse reaching the spinal cord is sent to the brain, it must cross over from one side to the other; most of the important impulse pathways cross in the midbrain. When returning to carry out their motor objectives—to stimulate muscles to contract—they must cross back again. If a body area affected by a brain lesion is supplied by nerves that have not crossed—specifically, the cranial nerves—the lesion will be found on the same side of the brain as the body manifestation. If the area is supplied by nerves that have crossed over, the lesion will be found on the side opposite the body manifestation. It should be obvious that its exact location must be determined by the symptoms it causes, especially if surgical therapy is contemplated. Because the brain is encased in the cranium (skull), a thick-walled box of bone, random search and manipulation are impossible.

The brain needs a constant supply of fresh blood. Functional damage to the brain cells causing loss of consciousness occurs within ten seconds of complete cardiac cessation. Because the heart rarely stops so abruptly and completely, complete deprivation is an unusual occurrence. Transient loss of consciousness may occur with partial deprivation. Structural cell damage occurs after about three minutes of brain ischemia, and cell death may be found after ten to twelve minutes of complete oxygen deprivation from either suffocation or vascular obstruction.

The brain is supplied with blood by four large arteries, two on each side. The internal carotid arteries ascend along the side of the neck and enter the skull through an opening in front of and deep to the ears. The two vertebral arteries ascend just behind the internal carotids, enter the skull, and join together to form the basilar artery. All of the numerous arteries that branch out and through the brain are outgrowths of the basilar or one of the two internal carotid arteries. Nature was farsighted enough to join these large supply arteries just after they enter the skull in a loop of vessels called the circle of Willis. This arrangement allows one of the main channels to close without necessarily damaging the brain. The closure of one of the branches of this arrangement, however, is more disastrous, because these vessels are the sole suppliers for their areas.

The blood supply to brain tissue can be jeopardized by a gradual closure of its supplier artery as the result of blood-clot formation (thrombosis) on an atheromatous plaque or by sudden closure resulting from a clot that has formed elsewhere and been carried in the blood stream to the brain (embolism). These emboli usually come from the heart, where clots were formed because of atheromatous damage. A third form of interference with the blood supply to the brain occurs when an artery bursts, called cerebral hemorrhage. This is a common finale to a long course of severe hypertension; it may also be precipitated by arterial weakening because of atherosclerosis. It is clear that whatever the mechanism of the vascular damage to the brain, atherosclerosis is an important culprit, as either a primary or secondary agent. Because it is not always possible to be certain which of the above mechanisms has caused the trouble, doctors avoid using the precise term and favor calling the process a cerebrovascular accident (CVA).

Of the three, the most common type of CVA is caused by thrombosis of an arterial vessel above the circle of Willis, the second most common is embolism of one of these vessels, and the third is rupture with hemorrhage, usually in association with high blood pressure. Although the symptoms may be quite similar whichever the cause, each cerebrovascular accident should be treated according to the mechanism that produced it.

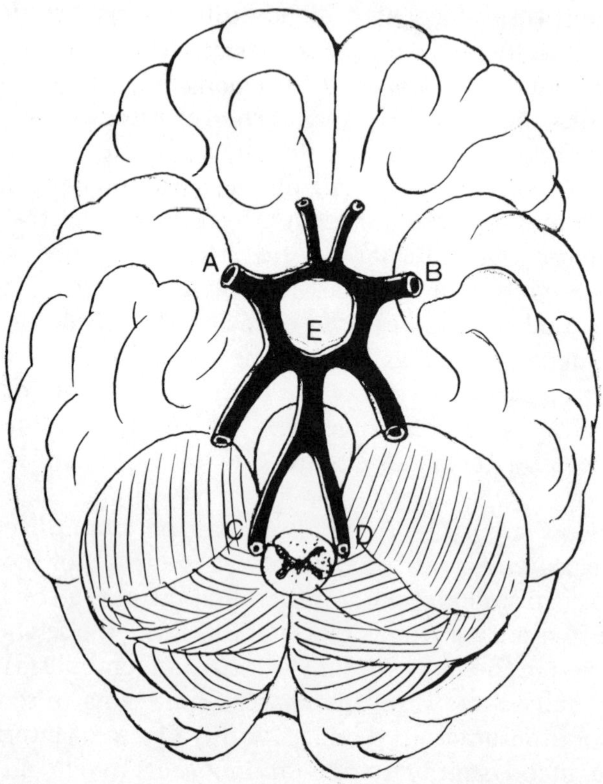

Circle of Willis, seen in view of the undersurface of the brain. (A and B) the right and left internal carotid arteries; (C and D) the right and left vertebral arteries. The brain's entire blood supply comes through these vessels. However, obstruction of one of these may be less damaging than closure of one of their smaller branches, because all four arteries feed the circle of Willis (E) and the other three healthy vessels may compensate for the obstructed fourth. Closure of any two of these vessels is always fatal.

It becomes important, therefore, for the physician to determine the exact cause. In all three mechanisms, brain tissue is destroyed and symptoms are registered in peripheral regions supplied by the nerves from the cells that have been damaged.

Paralysis of one or more groups of muscles is perhaps the most obvious and common manifestation of CVA. The muscles cannot contract although they are still healthy. They would contract as well as ever if they were supplied by the proper impulses. Bereft of impulses, they become flaccid and useless. Nature does not tolerate uselessness. If a muscle remains without its nerve supply for a protracted length of time, it wastes away. As the muscle cells deteriorate they are replaced by fibrous scar tissue. Scar tissue always contracts as it ages, so

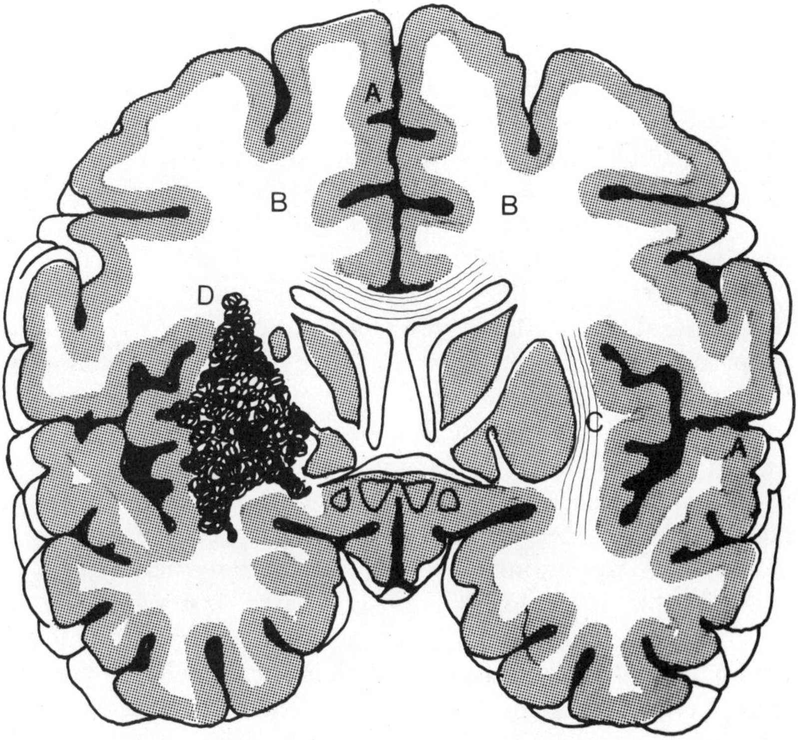

Cerebrovascular hemorrhage, seen in a section through the midportion of the brain from the rear. The left middle cerebral artery has ruptured in the region of the left internal capsule (C). This is the most common site of cerebrovascular accident. The mass of escaped blood (D) has destroyed the greater portion of a vital area of the left hemisphere, interrupting the nerve tracts to cause paralysis of the left side of the face and the right arm and leg. (A) gray matter; (B) white matter.

the muscle is permanently shortened; the resulting spasticity permanently distorts the affected area after a period of weeks or months.

Any muscle of the body can be involved. When one of the eye muscles becomes paralyzed, crossed eyes may develop, causing double vision. If the tongue or throat muscles are involved, the patient will have difficulty talking or swallowing. When face muscles are affected, one side of the face sags and there is loss of expression. All of these muscles are supplied by cranial nerves that have not crossed over, which means they will be encountered on the same side as the brain lesion.

When a skeletal muscle (one serving the arm or leg) is involved, the part becomes weakened or entirely limp and paralyzed. It remains flaccid for several weeks and then, if the impulses are not restored, spasticity and shortening of the muscle begin to develop. The arm will bend at the wrist and elbow into a permanent spastic position. If the leg is affected, it stiffens and is drawn toward the midline, becoming useless and even impeding locomotion. Part of the treatment for cerebrovascular accidents is the prevention of such muscle contracture by electrical stimulation and passive exercise.

Sensory nerve centers may also be involved. The manifestations of sensory paralyses are called agnosias and are specified by the sense involved. Visual agnosia means the prevention of proper registration of optic images; auditory agnosia is the distortion of hearing. Agnosia may be total, with resultant blindness or deafness, or may be partial, causing various types of distortion: apples may taste like onions, roses may smell like frying bacon. If the brain lesion is massive, it may involve all sensory intake and plunge the patient into coma; he may not regain consciousness. If he does, he has only about a 50 percent chance of surviving the attack and he is almost certain to have some residual paralysis.

Cerebrovascular accident occurs no more frequently in men than in women. It is most likely to strike those over sixty. Typically, the victim of a moderately severe CVA may have had a history of hypertension or of one or more transient ischemic attacks (TIA) with more or less complete recovery. If conscious, he may complain of double vision or his eyes may deviate toward the side of the brain lesion. His speech may be garbled or slurred. One eyelid may droop and that side of his face sag. The arm or leg on the opposite side may be numb and paralyzed.

The gravity of the situation depends upon the site of the lesion, its size, and its cause. When vital centers are involved, death may occur within minutes although this is quite unusual. Death from a cerebrovascular accident more commonly takes an hour or longer, although the symptoms develop in minutes. Massive destruction of motor areas of the brain may cause extensive paralysis but leave the patient's intellect completely untouched.

Transient ischemic attacks are not uncommon, but their mechanism and cause are poorly understood. There is apparently a cessation of blood supply in a localized area of the brain for a brief period of time. Unconsciousness or all the classic stroke symptoms may prevail for minutes or even hours. In the case of TIA, however, recovery is complete. The victim may suffer but one of these attacks or several, sometimes hundreds, but he will almost always eventually have a true stroke that will run the usual course and leave him with permanently faulty sensory or muscle functions.

TIAs may also appear in the form of "little strokes." Older people, particularly those with atherosclerosis or hypertension, may notice slight alterations in their motor capacities such as impaired coordination of one extremity, or perhaps alterations in sensory images. They may be troubled by peculiar smells that no one else notices or by changes in the intensity of sounds.

If the CVA patient survives for a day or two, symptom improvement is the rule. When the brain lesion is small, improvement may begin within hours and go on to complete recovery within twenty-four to forty-eight hours. The longer the delay before improvement is apparent, the less optimistic are the chances of recovery. If after ten days no evidence of recovery is apparent, we can expect little ever to occur. Lessening of paralysis and increase in strength, once started, may continue up to six months. After that there is apt to be no change, although improvement in speech and muscle coordination may continue for a year or even longer.

Prevention is the best treatment for cerebrovascular accident. Because the underlying cause in the great majority of these cases is atherosclerosis, every sensible precaution against that disease should be regarded as a vital necessity. The later chapters of this book will concern themselves with how to prevent atherosclerosis. And because hypertension has been implicated as a cause of cerebral hemorrhage, the third most common type of CVA, preventive treatment of hypertension is becoming part of routine health care.

In the past decade, great strides have been made in the improvement of physical therapy and rehabilitation of CVA patients. Much can be done today to get paralyzed cases back into the useful currents of society. Hospitals are being built to treat and take care of them. Progress has been a long time in coming but rehabilitation is proving itself to be worth every effort expended.

There is another type of intracranial hemorrhage, intracranial, though it is not intracerebral. This is ruptured saccular aneurysm of the cerebral arteries. Aneurysm of the aorta was discussed earlier as a complication of atherosclerosis. Aneurysms of the cerebral arteries are entirely different in their origin. They appear to be caused by a congenital weakness in the wall of the vessel that results in small blisterlike saccular protrusions of the arteries at the base of the brain before they enter the brain substance. The rudiments of these outpouchings may be present at birth, but they do not develop until later on in life, more rapidly in cases of hypertension. They may rupture at any time in adolescence or thereafter. This occurrence usually announces itself with sudden, violent headache. The patient often collapses and becomes unconscious. He may die within a matter of hours. The age incidence and the lack of localizing symptoms usually make the diagnosis obvious. Some cases can be treated successfully by surgery, but the mortality is high. About half of these patients die within six months, usually with recurrence.

One of the disconcerting and unhappy prospects of aging is caused by senile dementia, a brain disease in which a perfectly normal, intelligent person gradually loses his mental ability.

Although this is one of the most common ailments of the elderly, little is known about its cause and mechanism. This is a tragic irony in view of the fact that almost every family in this country has experienced or will at some time in the future experience the decline into senile dementia of a beloved relative.

The affected person, who may be greatly admired and highly intelligent, undergoes a change of personality; he becomes quarrelsome and suspicious, his intellectual capacity decreases until he is unable to read, write, or carry on a rational conversation. All the while he may remain in a state of glowing physical health.

Senile dementia is usually so insidious in onset that members of the family who see the patient every day may not be aware of its presence until it is fairly well advanced. Grandpa becomes forgetful of recent events but because this is such a commonplace happening among the elderly nothing much is thought of the matter. He may repeatedly recount the time that William Jennings Bryan came to town while stumping for the presidency, but he won't remember what was for breakfast this morning. This loss of memory for recent events worsens until he is unable to carry on a conversation because by the time he tries to finish a sentence he cannot remember what he started to say. Eventually he cannot remember his own name nor the faces of his intimate family. He is a helpless and dependent creature, occupied with the musings of the distant past that float like stray clouds across his consciousness.

Although there is little factual evidence to prove it, most investigators feel that a great preponderance of this type of intellectual deterioration in the aged is caused by a slowly progressive cerebral ischemia, the result of arteriosclerosis plus a failing general circulation compounded by atherosclerosis. Put all these elements together and we have a logical explanation if not a proven case.

I hope that this chapter has impressed you with the importance of the role that atherosclerosis plays in the diseases of the central nervous system. It is involved in about half of all the reasons for hospital admissions for neurological disorders, including admissions for tumors, infections, and trauma. Again I must emphasize that the term atherosclerosis is a sleeper. The layperson rarely uses it, despite the fact that more than half of us will die of one or more of its consequences. If we would all acknowledge that the cause of death in myocardial infarction is atherosclerosis, that the cause of death in most cases of stroke is atherosclerosis, and that senile dementia is hastened by atherosclerosis, then perhaps more of us would seriously consider what we could do to prevent this arterial deterioration.

9

Diet-related Diseases

In addition to the foregoing killing and crippling conditions, a number of other diseases caused or influenced by the food we eat are worth our attention. This book could not be considered complete without at least an acknowledgment of the more important of these and an explanation of how diet plays a role in their occurrence and progression.

One of the most common, yet perhaps the least talked about, is osteoporosis. Literally an increase in the porosity of the bones, this condition weakens the skeleton. It is much more common than most people imagine; indeed, most women after sixty suffer at least some of its symptoms, and it is almost as common in men over seventy. About a quarter of all people will reveal some x-ray evidence of this skeletal disease.

Osteoporosis is a major underlying cause of bone fracture in old people, and it interferes with bone healing, thus retarding or preventing recovery. The most common fracture in the aged occurs at the neck of the femur, the thigh bone. In fact, hip fracture is the third most common cause of death in old people, following closely behind the complications of atherosclerosis and cancer. It is usually taken for granted that the fracture is the result of a fall by a person made unsteady by old age. A close scrutiny is apt to show that the reverse is often the case: a sudden step downward or a twisting movement may place a sudden and unusual stress on a femur weakened by osteoporosis. The hip fractures from the stress and this causes the fall.

Because osteoporosis weakens all of the bones of the skeleton, symptoms may be widespread and general, but they are likely to be more severe when stress-bearing bones are involved. The femur is the site of the greatest stress, resulting in hip fracture. Next are the vertebrae, the bones of the spine, particularly those at the lower end of the spine which bear the greatest weight. A vertebra is shaped like a round block, a little higher (in the lower spine) than it is wide. When badly weakened by osteoporosis, it may collapse. This causes shortening of stature, bending of the spine, and pressure on the numerous nerves related to the spinal cord in the affected region. Pain may be felt in the lower back and it may radiate along the course of the damaged nerves, especially down the back of the legs.

The causes of osteoporosis (there are many and they are usually found in combination) are exceedingly complex. The strength of bone may be decreased when the soft bone matrix is not manufactured as fast as it is normally worn away, when the bone matrix is worn away at an abnormally rapid rate, or when there is a failure to deposit calcium and phosphorus in the matrix, which results in bone softening. Diminished secretion of sex hormones in the elderly may cause an increase in the rate of bone destruction. This condition is often called postmenopausal osteoporosis. When grandma takes to her rocking chair she reduces the exercise that supplies the stimulus for matrix formation. Old people frequently become picky about food and fail to eat the foods and minerals that provide the building blocks for bone formation. Because old people are often resigned to pains in the joints, they may suffer in silence while osteoporosis worsens and eventually threatens their lives.

Everyone over the age of fifty should take steps to reduce the probability of falling victim to this bone disease whose complications kill so many elderly people. An exercise routine should be maintained throughout life. The exercise need not be strenuous; walking or swimming will do very nicely. Diet should be carefully evaluated; it must contain plenty of precious proteins. The teeth must be kept in good repair so that a wide variety of meats can be eaten. Calcium and phosphorus intake must not be neglected. A glass of skimmed milk daily will supply the former, and adequate amounts of the latter will be supplied if meat is included in the diet. Trace amounts of fluorine probably help stabilize the mineralizing process. Vitamins, especially vitamin D, are of greater importance at this end of life than they are any time after childhood. Supplementary vitamins should be taken by most people over sixty. Finally, if there is evidence of osteoporosis even though the diet supplies adequate amounts of proteins, minerals, and vitamins and a good exercise program is followed, then the possibility of failing sex hormones or a more complicated bone disease must be considered. These are matters for a physician's attention.

Another common disease that is influenced by dietary intake is diabetes mellitus. Sugar does not cause "sugar diabetes," but it is all-important in its control. One of the symptoms of this disease, caused by an inability to metabolize carbohydrates properly, is urinary frequency. The word diabetes comes from the Greek "to pass through"; mellitus is derived from the Greek word for honey. Urinary frequency also occurs in diabetes insipidus, the cause of which is completely different. Because diabetes mellitus is common and diabetes insipidus rare, we are apt to consider only the former when diabetes is mentioned. People with diabetes must watch their sugar and fat consumption, because an inability to metabolize sugar (the problem in diabetes) affects utilization of fats. When a diagnosis of diabetes has been made, the diet must be prescribed by a physician; diabetics should not attempt to manage their own diets.

Hiatal hernia is a common abnormality in the digestive system, and one of the most frequent causes of indigestion. Any outpouching of a normal pathway is called a hernia. In this instance, the lower portion of the esophagus opens into the stomach through an opening in the diaphragm. If the diaphragm is poorly formed, this opening may be larger than normal. Because there is a positive pressure within the abdomen and a negative pressure within the chest, a pocket of the stomach wall is formed and slides up through the opening alongside the esophagus into the chest. Gastric acids are regurgitated into this pocket, causing a burning pain called water brash or heartburn. A high percentage of so-called acid indigestion is caused by such hiatal hernias, though many sufferers go through their entire lives without knowing the cause.

The symptoms of hiatal hernia may vary considerably depending upon the habits of those who suffer them. In those who retire shortly after eating, the symptoms usually appear between two and three hours after the last meal. For these people, the symptoms may be relieved if they change their position in bed, because turning may encourage drainage of the pocket by gravity. The pain is usually alleviated by neutralizing the gastric acidity; milk, sodium bicarbonate, or one of the extravagantly advertized commercial remedies will usually do the trick. Choose a compound that does not contain aspirin, which, it is believed, encourages bleeding from the inflamed gastric lining. Acid foods, such as orange juice, often bring on attacks of pain as may fatty foods, particularly greasy sauces, strong spices, and condiments (tabasco, horseradish, mustard), and undiluted alcoholic drinks.

The symptoms of hiatal hernia may be so similar to those of peptic ulcer that only upper gastrointestinal x-rays taken after the patient has swallowed barium may make the distinction. Frequently the acid within the hernial sac may cause ulceration.

Unfortunately, the repair of hiatal hernia through surgery is difficult, the chance of poor side effects relatively high, and the certainty of cure somewhat in doubt. Because hiatal hernia rarely has serious complications (occasionally it may cause serious hemorrhage), most people prefer to alter eating and other habits and learn to live with the symptoms they cannot prevent. With a bit of intelligent discipline, most are relatively successful.

Let us conclude this discussion with the counsel that you should know more than the usual household admonishments about the relation of the food you eat to the state of your health. As gourmet Anthelme Brillat-Savarin once wrote, "Tell me what you eat and I will tell you what you are."

I am afraid that the matter is somewhat overstated; it isn't that easy. I have tried to mention the most important among the numerous diseases related to diet, important because of their frequency. They are apt to affect most of us if we remain ignorant of their possibilities. However, none of the diseases that affects the gastrointestinal tract, not even diabetes and osteoporosis together, can compare in frequency and importance with atherosclerosis. The complications of atherosclerosis are the killers of mankind. We believe that at last we know enough about the mechanisms of this disease to do something in the way of prevention. Fat is our worst enemy and our most insidious one; atherosclerosis is caused in one way or another by fat, and it is fat that makes our food taste so good. Fat is the chief offender, but too much sugar, which must be converted into fat for storage, is bad too. Obesity is not only an esthetic curse; it is a disease. Cyril Connolly wrote, in *The Unquiet Grave*, "Imprisoned in every fat man a thin man is wildly signalling to be let out." For our appearance, our health, and our longevity, let us give him his freedom!

10

The Gastrointestinal Tract

This book is concerned with the diseases of man that are related to the food he eats. Not only should we be interested in the kinds of food that sustain us and those that do us harm, but we should also understand how our tissues utilize the nourishment that is given them. An important part of this process is digestion. An understanding of digestion is made easier if we can visualize the digestive tract and how it developed as it did.

The human body is essentially a tube, a vastly specialized and complicated one, but a tube nonetheless. When we contemplate the evolution of that marvelous machine, the human body, we see what nature has been up to all these years.

The formula for all living things is painfully simple: life equals competition. Every living thing, with the possible exception of a few human beings I know, competes constantly for its subsistence. Because man managed to grow a wondrously efficient knob of tissue at one end of his spinal cord, an organ that we call the brain, he has been able to beat the racket. But not by much and not for long.

I have insisted that all living things proliferate to the extent of their supply of nourishment. Food! Its attainment is the most important factor in life. It should not surprise us that nature has been preoccupied over the past several million years with improving the efficiency of our use of it. The species capable of adapting their equipment to the available supplies were the ones able to multiply. Those that could not adapt perished.

When the seething caldron of the earth had cooled sufficiently for the distillation of its vapors to fall back as water, the chemical brew on the earth's surface was diluted sufficiently to support living organisms. The earliest of these were composed of a single cell floating aimlessly in a concentrated sea. This cell took its nourishment from its environment, used what it needed, and cast away the waste. It was a simple life but not a very interesting one. Nature had more grandiose ideas.

Some cells became more proficient at doing certain things than others, and when two or more of these specialists merged, a single organism capable of performing a number of functions was produced. The goal, as far as we are concerned after four million years along the evolutionary path, was man. The first of innumerable problems along the way was caused by the isolation of those units that had become cell locked—that is, isolated from their supplies of food by the cells that grew around them. Rolling the mass of cells into a cylinder solved the problem by making it possible for the outside environment to flow through it and thus reach the previously inaccessible interior cells. That was the genesis of the gastrointestinal tract. Every species of living organism with only a few unimportant exceptions has been using it ever since.

As each species struggled to increase the efficiency with which it was able to utilize the nutrients available to it, the original tube was modified. The basic principle, however, was retained. The human gastrointestinal tract does not differ greatly from those of many of the lower forms. A course in comparative anatomy leaves one astonished at how similar are the intestinal tracts of man and the angleworm. Nature is an inveterate gambler and once the race is won, she has a tendency to lose interest. All the same, there are some splendid modifications in the human digestive tract that are important enough to deserve consideration.

To deal effectively with the materials that we are able to use as foods, this important system eventually was divided into seven connected segments, each modified to perform a special function. The first need was to reduce the raw food masses to a size that would not block the canal and would allow the various digestive juices access to all its parts. Food had to be torn apart and ground up, an impossible task for soft tissue to accomplish. An adroit grinding machine was the answer and, indeed, it is such an ingenious contraption that one must marvel at its existence. Hard, sharp blades and solid grinders had to be produced from soft tissue. This was accomplished by weaving a pliable matrix that has an affinity for crystalline salts. Osteoid tissue is the matrix. It is soft until it becomes impregnated with crystalline calcium phosphate, then it becomes as hard as stone and as rigid as steel. From this material nature fashioned dentine and enamel for the teeth and bone for the jaws which support and manipulate them. Hunks of food could thus be torn apart and ground up for swallowing. This segment of the digestive tract is the mouth.

The next portion of the alimentary canal, the pharynx, had to be devised to compensate for one of nature's blunders. Isolated cells within the organism need not only food but also oxygen, and they need a constant and continuous supply of it. In the lowest forms of life, the digestive and respiratory systems are separate and independent. Insects breathe through multiple narrow air tubules that penetrate into the interior of their bodies. That is why contact with a spreading agent such as a light oil (kerosene) causes them to suffocate. As we approach the higher forms, we can note nature's concern with maintaining a constant supply of oxygen. Obstruction of the single air inlet caused instant death in some species. Nature remedied that weakness by crossing the respiratory and digestive tracts and designing a double opening (nose and mouth) for the former. Like other of nature's solutions, it caused more problems than it solved. Air drawn into the food passage causes trouble for both men and race horses, and food lodged in the respiratory passage can be quite dangerous, even lethal. Nature patched this up as best she could by devising a flap valve (glottis) at the point where the two tracts cross.

The development of the respiratory system presented another difficulty. The simplest way to move air into and out of a tissue area is by means of a bellowslike mechanism. The chest is a simple and fairly efficient version. The interior space is enlarged by elevating the curved, rigid supports (ribs) and lowering the floor (diaphragm). When you inhale, the space is enlarged and the air rushes in. When you exhale, you relax the muscles that accomplish this action and the space is diminished. All this could be accomplished with less risk of mishap were it not that the first portion of the alimentary and respiratory systems cross. Some way had to be devised to get the food into the abdomen, the area in which it is processed, without interfering with the bellows action of the chest. The simplest solution would have been to place the food inlet (the mouth) nearer the food-processing plant; say, in the abdominal wall—less esthetic, perhaps, but certainly more direct. Nature chose instead to modify a segment of the digestive tract to transport food through the bellows. We call this segment the esophagus; it has no purpose other than to serve as a conduit.

The stomach is an expanded saclike organ between the esophagus and the intestine. Because the need at this level of the digestive tract is to mix and homogenize the various food constituents and to stir in several digestive juices, the stomach must be large enough to contain a considerable volume of food at one time. It must be capable of coordinated rhythmic contractions so that it can mix and churn its contents. It must be fitted with an inlet valve to keep its contents from being regurgitated into the esophagus, and an outlet valve to keep them from escaping into the intestine before they have been thoroughly mixed. The stomach is housed in the abdomen, a cavity which lies midway between the chest and the pelvis.

The stomach secretes four juices that are essential for proper digestion. Each is manufactured by specially modified cells forming the membrane that lines the stomach cavity. One of these juices is an enzyme called pepsin, which breaks down proteins into its simpler constituents, polypeptides. It can do this only in an acid medium. Nature obliged by specializing cells to secrete hydrochloric acid, the second digestive juice. But hydrochloric acid injures the other cells of the stomach lining, so a third type of cell was devised to manufacture mucus, a protective coating substance. To make sure that this complicated sequence was not all in vain, another enzyme, gastrin, was compounded by a fourth cell type. The gastrin cells are found in the upper portion of the stomach lining. When food enters the stomach and stretches the upper portion of the wall, it triggers the secretion of gastrin, which in turn stimulates the pepsin cells to secrete. It also signals the pancreas to begin its work, and the gall bladder to empty a quantity of bile into the duodenum in preparation for the food that is about to follow. When the meal has been thoroughly churned, the outlet valve opens and the stomach contents begin to drain into the duodenum.

The physician calls the intestine the gut, a good old Anglo-Saxon word that means just what it says. The gut is divided into four parts: the duodenum, the small intestine, the large intestine or colon, and the rectum. Each segment has been modified for special function.

The duodenum is a short, C-shaped segment about twelve inches (30.5cm) long. From its lining membrane the two most important and complex abdominal organs, the liver and the pancreas, develop in the human embryo. Although these organs have adopted other important body functions, a review of comparative anatomy reveals that they were originally conceived to aid in the digestive process.

The liver is the body's largest single organ. It supplies the digestive tract with bile, a complicated solution of salts, pigments, and cholesterol, which emulsifies fat so that it can be acted upon by other digestive juices. Manufactured by the liver, bile is stored in the gall bladder, a saclike structure attached to the underside of the liver. The gall-bladder wall is formed of contractile muscles that force the bile into the duodenum through an opening close to the opening of the pancreatic duct.

The pancreas was devised as the principal source of digestive enzymes. It produces three, one for each food type. One kind of cell secretes amylase, which splits the more complicated starches and polysaccharides into simple sugars so that they can be absorbed through the intestinal wall and utilized by the cells. Other cells produce lipase, which breaks down the emulsified fats into their constituent fatty acids, glycerides, and glycerol. A third enzyme, trypsin, is produced to split the polypeptide constituents of protein into their component amino acids.

Food is ingested in the pharynx, transposed through the chest by the esophagus, mixed in the stomach, and then treated by digestive enzymes in the duodenum. It must now be separated into nutrients and wastes, the former to be absorbed, the latter to be stored and eventually excreted. Most of the absorption takes place in the small intestine.

Effectiveness of absorption depends upon two factors: the permeability and the surface area of the absorbing membrane. The intestinal wall is considerably more than a colander. Nature has augmented the physical aspects of absorption by specializing the cells in the membrane of the small intestine to work actively. Materials are selected from the intestinal contents and taken into the lining cells by physiological processes that require the expenditure of energy. Achieving the maximum surface for this important step in the digestive process requires a very long passageway. The immense surface is achieved with the great length of the small intestine, over twenty feet (6m). To accommodate this structure without endowing us with the physique of a python, nature ingeniously folded the small intestine into complicated loops. Movement of the intestinal contents was achieved by a wall composed of circular muscles that contract rhythmically to produce peristaltic waves. These waves push the contents along, not too slowly (if they did, the result would be constipation) and not too rapidly (which would result in diarrhea).

The large intestine is considerably shorter than the small intestine but it has a larger diameter. By the time the food reaches this portion of the digestive tract, most of the valuable constituents have been removed and utilized. The lining cells of the large intestine are less specialized than those of the small intestine, but the mechanical aspects of absorption can be carried out here. This is the site for the absorption of large amounts of fluids. The far end of the colon, the rectum, acts as a storage site for wastes to allow their disposal at times and places of convenience.

Man has come a long way from the days when he was forced to spend practically all his time and energy in procuring food. Or has he? You might be surprised if you stopped to add up the amount of time and energy spent in earning the money required to buy your food, the energy necessary for its preparation, the time allotted for its consumption. And yet few people know and understand how we process the nutritional elements in our environment to supply the energy required for the lives we want to live. Perhaps this ignorance lies at the root of the two distressing complications of improper food consumption, obesity and atherosclerosis.

Thoughtful people in centuries past have attempted to understand the problems consequent to poor eating habits. From the beginning of time, medicine men enhanced their reputations with their dietary and therapeutic recommendations. Strip away the sentimental romance that people employ in describing these, and the occasional coincidences of real value, and there is very little left. One of the earliest attempts at a rational approach to the investigation into the physiology of digestion occurred during the seventeenth century, carried out by a Frenchman named René de Reayer. A bird fancier, he saw his pets regurgitate undigestible materials they had eaten—feathers, fur, and small bones. He fed them pieces of sponge and when these were regurgitated he was able to analyze the fluids they had absorbed. He found that these fluids acted on meat outside the stomach in a way that resembled digestion. In this manner he first established the significance and function of the stomach's digestive enzymes.

One of the most dramatic episodes in the research of digestive physiology was carried out by an American army surgeon in the early part of the nineteenth century. William Beaumont encountered a young Canadian woodsman who had been shot in the abdomen. When the wound healed it left a passageway between the stomach and the exterior. Beaumont was able to extract and analyze the gastric contents of the man's stomach at various stages of digestion. He thus discovered the role of hydrochloric acid in digestion.

Claude Bernard, a nineteenth-century Frenchman, is generally credited with being the father of physiology. He investigated the manner in which foods are broken down and how they provide energy for cell maintenance and growth. Today, physiologists, chemists, and metabolists, devoting their energies and great amounts of research endowment, have amassed vast scientific knowledge that has made life more pleasant and healthful and lengthened its expectancy. Those who appreciate this great work are apt to be impatient with the natural food faddists who preach their views from a store of ignorance. We should also be impatient with those who ignore the opportunity to acquaint themselves with this knowledge so readily available, knowledge so vital to health and longevity.

Armed with an understanding of the anatomy and function of the gastrointestinal tract, we can now turn our attention to what happens when we fail to use these endowments to our best advantage. Obesity is the most common result of such indiscretion, as we shall see in the succeeding chapter.

11

Obesity, a Disease

I have stated that in nature's order of things, all organisms live to the capacity of their environment. This can be expressed as a simple equation: the quantity of living things always equals the quantity of food available to nourish them. Wildlife multiplies in the good years that burgeon with foliage and seeds; it diminishes in the barren years. It is not that animals are better fed in a good year than in a bad one. The equation always holds: in the good year there are more animals as well as more food. The result of this arrangement is that most organisms in the wild state are almost always hungry, and those whose food is abundant and acquired without competition—that is, those that are fed by man—are all too often fat. Hunger is a driving motive next in importance to the reproductive urge.

Nature does not always distinguish between those at the top of her order (man, as we like to think) and those beneath them. In order to maintain his physiology in tone and pitch, man should exist in a state of mild hunger; at least, nature intended it thus. In those who have learned to discipline their appetites, obesity is never a problem. The rest of us prefer to find a way that is more fun.

Weight is solely a matter of calories. Other explanations cannot be considered valid; there are simply no data that will support them. I am willing to entertain the possibility that the alimentary canal of one person may be less efficient in absorbing nutrients than that of another, but I know of no statistical data to support this hypothesis. Anyway, it is still a matter of calories. I am not including those instances in which obvious disease affects the gut. Those people languish and grow thin because they lack the effective mechanisms of getting nutrient materials from their intestinal tracts into their tissues. I am referring to the mistaken hypothesis that some people accomplish this business with greater efficiency than others, an easy explanation that has nothing more than rationalization to support it.

There probably is a group, very small in number, in whom cerebral controls over appetite function abnormally. Neuroanatomists have found that in the outer portion of the hypothalamus, an area of the brain, there are centers that are activated when body tissues need food. When these centers are in operation we say that we have an appetite. In the inner portions of the hypothalamus are located other centers that counteract these appetite stimuli and give us a feeling of satiation. When these two centers are in functional balance, we find food palatable as long as our tissues are in need of nourishment, and quite the opposite when they are adequately supplied. If something were to go wrong in these two centers we would experience uncontrollable hunger continuously and stuff ourselves until we could not down another morsel. Obviously this would result in gross obesity, and just as obviously this rare cerebral lesion is not the cause of *your* weight problem.

The cause of obesity, in whatever form it appears, is the ingestion of more calories than the tissues can use up. The excess is stored as fat. In perhaps 99 percent of the cases, the cause of overeating is ignorance or lack of discipline. I know of no objective test that will delineate those with abnormal hypothalamic control, but the chances against that contingency are so great that you had best disregard it except as a final and desperate resort for an explanation. You should expect weight reduction to be uphill all the way. No one has ever invented a method that does not require forbearance and self-discipline.

Then must we be sentenced to a life of eternal hunger? To be perfectly honest, yes. However, it isn't quite as bad as all that.

Even before man came down from the trees, he was occupied with finding ways to best nature. When his environment became uncomfortably cold or wet, he invented shelter. When he encountered competitors that could run faster and fight more fiercely than he, he invented speedier means of locomotion and weapons more deadly than any nature could devise. When his health was threatened by outside elements such as infections, he developed a complicated mass of knowledge, techniques, and curative chemicals (we call their aggregate the science of medicine) to counter them.

It is only natural that man should try to beat hunger pangs. He soon learned their causes; they are not obvious. The sensation of satiety depends only partially upon the sheer bulk of the content of the stomach. We have come to believe that when the stomach is empty it growls, and we interpret this bit of anatomical gauchery as a signal that it is time to find forage. In fact, it usually is not the stomach that growls, and the phenomenon has very little to do with the sensation of hunger. The noise originates in the small and large intestines, where gas within the tract is propelled noisily around bends by especially strong contractions of the muscles that encircle the gut wall. Doctors call this phenomenon borborygmus, a fascinating term that has onomatopoeic origins.

The uncomfortable sense of bulk within the stomach was probably invented by nature to let the animal know when it had had enough to eat. We are told that gluttonous Romans emptied their stomachs by regurgitating in order to prolong their banquets. There is clearly more than the mass of stomach content in the complicated mechanism we call appetite. The endocrine glands secrete hormones directly into the blood stream, which carries them directly to their sites of action, the cells. When the concentration of a vital substance needed by the cells falls to a critically low level, the endocrine glands secrete hormones that in turn affect cells at widely separated areas in the body but particularly in the brain. These sense-perception areas give rise to the sensations that we call hunger. There are many different kinds of hunger sensations: low blood sugar causes the feeling of faintness, a low sodium level results in the sensation of thirst, a low calcium level generates a feeling of tiredness. These mechanisms dictate much of our primary behavior. When the signal is given, the animal is sent off in search of food or drink or whatever it lacks.

The acquisition, preparation, digestion, absorption, and utilization of food is a complicated business, as any metabolist will readily assure you. It is within this chain of events that man has found his solace from hunger pangs. Nature keeps the animals of the lower orders in trim shape by limiting their food by adjusting their population to the food supply. But man, always eager to outdo nature, has guaranteed his environment against food shortage. In most parts of this hemisphere there is no such thing as an absolute food shortage. Man can eat as much as he wants of whatever he likes whenever he pleases—as long as he can pay for it. In arranging this convenience he has thrown a basic natural law out of balance. The result? Most of us are too fat for our own good.

Weight standards (and tables) vary, depending on the society we live in. The first weight tables were computed on the basis of the actual weights of large numbers of citizens. But if the entire population of a country is too heavy for its best health, these tables cannot be recommended as proper guides. Americans as a people have always been too heavy for their own good. The tables given in this book reflect a sane estimate of optimum weight. They may seem impossibly light to you; you will just have to adjust to reality. Rationalization rarely works in dietary matters.

In the roughest kind of generalization, if you are thirty years old and your weight is normal your life expectancy is around seventy-two years. For each four pounds you are overweight, you lose about one year of life. For example, if you are fifty pounds overweight during your youth and middle age you may expect to live only to around age sixty. These are hard figures and you may choose to believe that they do not apply to you. Don't count on it.

Most people do not maintain the weight that is most apt to promote their best health without some effort. This maintenance usually requires some knowledge of caloric values and the optimum proportions of the three basic food constituents: protein, fat, and carbohydrate. In the next several chapters I shall provide data to help you acquire eating habits that should promote good health.

12

The Nature of Food

Before we examine the character of the various types of substances that we use as foods, we should know what is meant by the terms calorie and metabolism.

A calorie (more correctly, a kilogram calorie) is that amount of energy required to raise the temperature of one kilogram of water (one liter, a little over a quart) one degree centigrade, from 14.5 degrees to 15.5, at atmospheric pressure. It is a fairly simple matter to calculate the number of calories in any oxidizable substance by burning it in a calorimeter and measuring the amount of heat that it produces. Metabolists have been busy for years measuring the caloric content of practically everything that can be classified as food.

Tissues use calories through the process of metabolism. Ingested food is broken down into its simplest constituents, taken into the cell, and oxidized (burned) by means of the cell's enzymes to form carbon dioxide, water, and wastes, which are carried away in the blood stream. Some of the carbon dioxide and water is used elsewhere in living tissues and some given off by the lungs. We exhale carbon dioxide and excrete water as vapor through the lungs, as sweat through the skin, and urine through the kidneys. Each of the trillion or more cells of our bodies is, in itself, a microscopic cosmos composed of millions of molecules, and each molecule has a specific atomic anatomy. The spatial relationship of these various atomic groups is such that an astonishing variety of chemical reactions can take place simultaneously and independently within the microscopic bit of tissue delineated by the cell wall. The cell, a structure too small to be seen with the naked eye, is a miniature chemical factory. Each cell acts as a unit, but it cooperates with millions of identical cells to perform a single physiological function. The various functions are then coordinated into organs such as the liver, the organs into systems such as the gastrointestinal system, and finally the systems into the body as a whole.

Most cells can burn only that amount of food that they need at the moment of activity. That is to say, food consumption is controlled by the metabolic rate of the cells concerned. Because all motion is accomplished by muscle contraction, it follows that much of our energy is expended by our muscle cells. But we also use energy in generating body heat, and the various steps in metabolism itself may require energy from an outside source to set it in motion.

There are five major components of the foods necessary for the growth and maintenance of tissues: proteins, carbohydrates, fats, vitamins, and minerals. The metabolism of the last two is rather complicated, so an abbreviated discussion of the subject will be reserved for the end of this chapter.

Proteins are the most vital of our foodstuffs. Amino acids combine in various groupings to form long chains called polypeptides. Polypeptides are then combined to produce proteins. As soon as the proteins reach the small intestine, they are partially broken down by the digestive processes, particularly by enzymes produced in the pancreas. These halfway products are absorbed by the cells lining the gastrointestinal tract and passed on directly into the venous blood stream. The blood carries them to the liver, which serves as the body's kitchen. It is here that our foodstuffs are processed for cellular consumption elsewhere in a manner analogous to that in which raw meats and vegetables are processed in our kitchens for consumption in our dining rooms. The liver returns the prepared nutrients to the blood, which then transports them to the body cells where they are used. These simple protein constituents are absorbed through the cell membranes; within the cell, they enter into the complicated process of metabolism.

Proteins supply the building material for new cells and the replacement of worn out cells. They are especially important for growing children, pregnant women, lactating mothers, and in the healing of extensive wounds, especially widespread burns, all of which require large amounts of protein nourishment.

Amino acids, the basic elements of proteins, are also important constituents of antibodies, which play such an important role in the body's defenses. Antibodies are produced in response to stimulation by an antigen, an invading or foreign protein substance such as pollen, the juices of certain foliage such as poison ivy and poison oak, insect toxins, and snake venom. When these chemical substances come in contact with our tissues, they cause the cells of our defensive system to make antibodies. Each antibody neutralizes a specific antigen. Antibodies are made from globulin, a protein substance found in blood plasma and prepared in the liver as a part of its metabolic routine. Globulin is converted into a specific antibody by the plasma cells found throughout the body. When disturbances occur in a given area, an allergy or a state of hypersensitivity may result. It follows, therefore, that most allergy-producing substances are proteins.

Proteins are compounded with carbohydrates to form mucopolysaccharides, the important constituents of the supportive substance between cells. Proteins compounded with lipids (fats) form lipoproteins, which play such an important role in atherosclerosis. Protein molecules are the largest of any of our foodstuffs. As I mentioned in Chapter 4, when lipoproteins are made up mostly of protein, the size of the particle is large and the density high, hence the term high-density lipoprotein (HDL). When the complex consists mostly of fat, the size of the particle is smaller and the density less: low-density lipoproteins (LDL).

Most of our ingested protein is used up during metabolic activity. The only manner in which proteins can be stored is if new cells are produced or the size of already existing cells, such as muscle, is increased. Within the living cells most of the protein is in the form of either ribo- or deoxyribonucleic acid (RNA or DNA). When the body is in desperate need of nutrition it can eat itself; that is, it can use cells for vital energy. It never does this except when available energy (carbohydrates) or stored energy (fats) is unavailable.

Although most protein is used up in metabolism, few proteins are burned up completely in the process. They are broken down into their constituent polypeptides, or sometimes further, into amino acids. Some of these are not usable by the tissues and so are reconstituted as urea, which is then excreted by the kidneys. Protein provides us with about 4.1 calories per gram.

Carbohydrate is the generic name for sugars and starches. Sometimes alcohols are included in this category as well. Carbohydrates—the name means carbon and water—are composed of atoms of carbon, hydrogen, and oxygen bound together in rings of six carbon atoms each. Each carbohydrate is made up of one or more rings. The simplest sugar, called a monosaccharide, has one ring; a disaccharide has two. Polysaccharides, such as starches, are composed of combinations of more than two rings. The alcohols, ethyl (drinking alcohol) and methyl (wood alcohol), consist of a fragment of a single ring. Carbohydrates must be broken down into the simple one-ring forms by the digestive processes before they can be utilized in cell metabolism. They are absorbed through the intestinal lining as monosaccharides and, like amino acids, are delivered directly into the venous blood stream and transported to the liver to be prepared for cell use. Carbohydrates serve as our immediate source of energy. They supply about the same amount of energy per gram as proteins, approximately 4.1 calories.

When metabolized, most of the carbon atoms are oxidized (burned), giving off energy; some are reconstituted with oxygen to form carbon dioxide, which is carried to the lungs by the red blood cells. There it is exhaled. The remaining oxygen and hydrogen atoms are combined to make water, excesses of which are excreted by the kidney as urine.

When more carbohydrates are ingested than can be used in immediate energy expenditure, the excess cannot be stored in unaltered form. It must first be broken down into its molecular constituents and then reassembled into fats for storage. Thus some of the objectives of a low-fat diet may be defeated by eating excessive amounts of sugars and starches.

The living organism was designed to eat when food is available, sometimes regularly, but more often with varying periods when no food is to be had. Living, however, requires a continuous expenditure of energy. Nature had to devise a system whereby energy could be stored in periods of excess to be used in periods of need. Fat is the answer to this problem. It is only because man has tampered with nature's ordinances by allowing himself more food than he needs that we have the problem of obesity. Wild animals, foraging for themselves, rarely become too fat.

The fat cell is a curious unit of tissue composition. It is a rather primitive connective-tissue cell that has become specialized to store fat. To accomplish this chore efficiently it grows to a huge size, many times larger than any other body cell, as the fat collects inside its membrane. In large aggregates these cells form masses of blubber. These masses require blood and so add to the work of the heart. Furthermore, they increase the body weight and so require greater work on the part of the body musculature, which in turn increases the burden on the heart. They occupy space and get in the way of the efficient functioning of vital organs.

Fat is our biggest dietary problem. Fat is the food substance of which we must be most careful, not only the concentrated fats such as lard, butter, cream, and egg yolks, but also the fat that is masked in fine dispersion about the muscle fibers in meats. Some meats—pork, duck, and goose—contain more fat than others, but there are also large quantities in beef (even lean beef) and lamb. Fat contains over twice the calories, about 9.2, per gram of either protein or carbohydrate, and even worse, it supplies the components that form the plaques that plug the arteries to our hearts (causing heart attack), our brains (causing stroke), our kidneys (causing high blood pressure), and our feet and toes (causing gangrene) in that most common of all deadly diseases, atherosclerosis.

Abnormal accumulations of fat represent one of nature's blunders, a failure to provide an efficient check in the necessary storage of energy. Health maintenance requires that each individual supply this check for himself. He can do it by limiting calorie intake or by providing sufficient energy expenditure. A combination to create an energy balance is the most sensible objective.

Fat consists of complex combinations of fatty acids. Some of these combinations are saturated with hydrogen, in which case they are called neutral fats. Others remain unsaturated and are free to combine with other chemical elements within the cells, particularly proteins. Such combinations make up cholesterol, triglyceride, and phospholipid components of our tissues. Among the phospholipids are the lipoproteins. As we know, the low-density lipoproteins (LDL) play an important role in atherosclerosis. We know also that the different fat-protein combinations in blood vary greatly in molecular size, and it now appears that it is size and density, rather than degree of saturation per se, that is important in the disturbances of fat metabolism.

When eaten, fat is emulsified in the upper intestine by bile from the liver and then broken down into fatty acids by the enzyme lipase provided by the pancreas. Fatty acids can be absorbed through the intestinal wall but not into the blood stream, as amino acids and sugars can. Instead, the fatty acids are collected by a special system, the lacteals, that carry lymph. This fat-laden lymph is shunted around the liver before it is sent into the general circulation. Nature has her reasons, devious as they sometimes seem. In this case, the fat-laden lymph does not pass through the liver because the liver cannot handle excess fats efficiently, particularly when its cells have been damaged by such toxins as alcohol. However, once excess fat is in the blood stream, it is carried through the heart and lungs and then is returned to the liver. This fat collects within the liver cells, which seem unable to get rid of it. The presence of abnormal amounts of fat enlarges the cells and interferes with their function. Eventually they may die and be replaced by fibrous connective tissue. This is one of the reasons why cirrhosis (fibrous scarring of the liver) and chronic alcoholism are so frequently associated.

Fat is our means of storing energy, but even if we had no need of stored energy we would still need fatty acids, because they are used in the formation of such vital compounds as hormones. When a problem develops in the metabolism of fats, ketones are formed. These products of incomplete breakdown of fat cannot be adequately excreted by the kidneys. It is the presence of abnormal amounts of ketones that causes most of the troubles in diabetes. Insulin plays an important role in the metabolism of fat, and diabetics must watch the amount of fats in their diets as well as the amount of carbohydrates.

Obesity, like diabetes, is a disturbance in fat metabolism. But in the great majority of the cases, there is no physiological reason for the metabolic problem. We usually bring it upon ourselves through ignorance, lack of motivation, or a willful disregard for the rules of health. The only sensible therapy is preventive, and for this we must maintain an energy balance. Caloric intake must equal caloric expenditure. Herein lie the two important variables, diet and exercise, that must be regulated. Frequently, nature does it for us. If she does not, each individual must. With the simple knowledge outlined in this book, the methods are easy to understand. Satisfactory fulfillment, however, may not be quite as easy to execute.

And vitamins? Vitamin pills are easy to take and relatively inexpensive. They usually are not necessary, but they save trouble in menu planning. So why not? It would be difficult for the average American adult to be deficient in the fat-soluble vitamins A and D, but it is possible to dose oneself with toxic amounts of these drugs. It is not uncommon, on the other hand, to develop shortages of the water-soluble vitamins (certain constituents of the B-complex and vitamin C) with diets that appear fairly normal. This is particularly true in those who drink alcoholic beverages. There is no danger here of toxic effects from large amounts of these vitamins, because excesses are eliminated in sweat and urine.

The American public spends a great deal of money each year to buy nothing of value, only lining the pockets of a number of very clever "professionals" who usually call themselves doctors. Almost none of them holds a doctorate of medicine and they are professional only in their knowledge and technique as salespeople. They prey on the public's ignorance. They sell wondrous combinations of vitamins, minerals, diet "extracts," herbs, "natural foods," and advice to a vast audience that can ill-afford their worthless products. They crowd every medium that will allow them space and time—ad columns in the press, television and radio programs. Their facade is one of dignity and concern for your welfare; their motive is the extraction of money from your pocket, and for a valueless product to boot. The average American on a typical American diet needs none of their wares, and if he did, he should be consulting a physician who understands these needs.

Most knowledgeable metabolists discourage the use of the vast majority of these nostrums, particularly herbs and minerals. It is probable that our tissues can occasionally profit by a booster or two among the vitamins. Why not take a sensible amount of B-complex and plenty of vitamin C, without necessarily believing a word that Linus Pauling says. You might also throw in a modest amount of vitamin E (high doses can be toxic) although no one knows what it does. I have a dear friend approaching ninety who is convinced that it "slows the aging process." In her case, something certainly has, and who wants to gamble with the fates on a matter so important and so personal?

13

The Balanced Diet

A balanced diet has little to do with the state of equilibrium, weight determination, or any of the other dictionary terms that are used to define the word *balance.* A balanced diet seems to be whatever combination of foods its proponent advocates; and license, rather than restraint, appears often to have been the guiding principle. Everyone is interested in what he eats and almost everyone is eager to give advice on the matter. All agree that a balanced diet is a combination of the three basic nutrients—proteins, carbohydrates, and fats—together with vitamins and essential minerals. Beyond this there is little accord.

Most of the argument has been concerned with the three principal elements, particularly in regard to weight loss. The public seems at last to have learned that pure protein diets, pure carbohydrate diets, and pure fat diets are not healthy diets. The exact ratios of these three factors to best ensure health, vigor, and maintenance of satisfactory weight have not been uniformly established. A review of a number of sources reveals that the diet of the average American is in a ratio somewhere near the following: proteins, 15 percent; carbohydrates, 45 percent; fats, 40 percent. If I could be sure that a person on a diet with this ratio were in perfect health, that his weight was satisfactory, and that his aorta contained no trace of atherosclerosis, I would be the first to say that this is the diet of choice. I would be willing to wager, however, that this person is not in perfect health, that he is at least a few pounds overweight, and that his arterial system is well on its way to destructive atherosclerosis. It will be many years before we know the ultimate truth. Most of us cannot wait.

If I were the least overweight I would strive for a nutrient ratio of 40 percent protein, 35 percent carbohydrate, and 25 percent fat. To some this will seem extreme. For those who can manage it, I will predict a life expectancy long beyond the average. Just as important, those who can maintain such a diet will remain as bright and intelligent up until their deaths as they were during their prime.

It is clear that the change I am advocating lies in switching the amounts of proteins and fats, increasing the former and decreasing the latter. To understand what such diet manipulation means, we should review the functions of each dietary constituent.

Proteins are used to replace worn-out cells and to build new ones. They are especially needed by growing children, pregnant and lactating women, in the healing of burns and extensive wounds (accidental or surgical), and in convalescence after debilitating disease. Each gram of protein provides about 4.1 calories. Carbohydrates are the source of the energy expended within twenty-four to forty-eight hours of consumption. If more carbohydrates are ingested than is necessary to satisfy this need, the excess is broken down and reconstituted as fat, which is then stored. A gram of carbohydrate has about the same caloric value as a gram of protein. Fat has a number of functions in the body, but its principal purpose is to provide a constant store of energy so that the body is capable of expending energy whenever the occasion demands. When partially broken down into its constituent fatty acids, fat combines with carbon from carbohydrates and polypeptides from proteins into a number of complex chemical substances, some of which are excreted, others used in normal physiology, and some, unfit for either of these, collect as unwanted lipid debris. It is this debris that may be deposited in the walls of our arteries, producing atherosclerosis.

Fats are the bête noir of the obese. They are the most important bearer of the flavors that make food tempting, and each gram provides 9.2 calories, about twice the calories of either proteins or carbohydrates.

In discussing the foods that serve no good purpose in our diets, we should keep in mind the food types and their caloric values. Proteins are the most valuable and perhaps the most interesting. We have already stated that proteins are constituted of combinations of twenty-six different amino acids. Ten of these are absolutely essential for tissue health. Eggs, meats, poultry, and fish contain these essential amino acids, along with a wide variety of others that are less essential but that do provide calories. Most vegetables are low in or lack proteins. The notable exceptions are all kinds of beans except string beans (the pod rather than the seed of the string bean is eaten). The caloric content of most vegetables in which the pod (snow peas), flesh (cucumbers, squash, cantaloupe), or stalk or leaf (celery and lettuce) are eaten is low. Peas, like beans, have a high protein content and a rather high caloric value. The trouble with vegetables as a protein source is that, except for soybeans, they lack one or more of the essential amino acids. Providing a sufficient quantity of proteins for health requires a large volume and variety.

There are a number of food substitutes available today whose only merit is that they reduce the number of calories in our diets. Most calorie-saving devices are found in two areas: low-calorie sweeteners to replace sugars and clever chemical manipulations of vegetable oils and synthetic fatty acids to simulate butter and animal fat. Saccharin is probably the oldest and best known of the low-calorie sweeteners. It would still be an admirable substitute for sugar if the research metabolists could make up their minds whether or not it is carcinogenic in humans. The so-called diet drinks owe their popularity to the fact that they contain low-calorie sweeteners instead of sugar. If one must drink soda pop, these are acceptable substitutes for the sugar-packed originals.

When butter became unobtainable during World War II, margarine broke through a barrier of prejudice that had theretofore repressed its use. With experience, manufacturers have adjusted taste, color, and consistency to fool the taste buds. And they have done so successfully. During the war on saturated fats, margarine, with less saturated fats than the butter it imitates, rose to a status of respectability and even dignity. Yet it has the same number of calories as butter. Then our weight-conscious chemists produced an "imitation" margarine with about half the calories of "real" margarine. Eventually, an imitation of an imitation has come to replace a fat once considered indispensable in the enjoyment of a decent meal. It serves its purpose although it does take a bit of adjustment in taste.

If you are to diet for weight reduction, you should be interested enough in the subject to commit to memory a short list of foods that should be eaten as infrequently as possible. Indeed, you should memorize two lists; both can be found in Chapter 18. One is of foods that are high in calories but of little nutritional importance; the second is of those that are high cholesterol formers, hereafter designated C-F. The latter are almost always high in calories too, so they are the worst offenders.

Foods that are high calorie and high C-F are the worst of all. They are lard, saturated oils, and butter. There are 125 calories in one tablespoon of oil, melted lard, or butter. One tablespoon of any one of these substances contains almost as many calories as two slices of bread. You may double the caloric value of a food simply by frying it, especially by deep-frying. The ramifications of this fact are far-reaching. The simplest way to cook many foods—eggs, meats, batter cakes—is to fry them. Deep-frying makes a special delight of vegetables such as potatoes, eggplant, and onions, but deep-fried foods are among the most important things you should learn to forego because of their caloric content and C-F character. Actually, foods fried in any fashion should be avoided whenever possible. This precaution observed, a giant step will have been taken.

There is an alternative to frying, not perfect, but it will do. A coating of lecithin—a complex of phosphorus, glycerol, and fatty acids usually derived from plant materials, can be used to prevent foods from sticking to the pan. Lecithin is not absorbed by the intestine so it has neither calories nor C-F properties. It is available in spray cans under several brand names. Sprayed over the surface of the utensil to be used and in some instances the food itself, this substance does not impart the flavor that frying gives, but it performs the main function of oils; it keeps food from sticking to the pan in which it is cooked.

Oils are one of the chief constituents of salad dressings and mayonnaise. You can cut down the C-F properties of these condiments by using the more unsaturated vegetable oils (corn, safflower, and soybean) in preference to palm or peanut oil, for example. Vegetable oils may be cut by one quarter with pure mineral oil to reduce their caloric values. (Buy oil labeled heavy or extra heavy; whether brand name or generic, it is all the same.) Mineral oil can be tolerated physiologically only in small quantities such as I recommend, but because it is not absorbed it has neither caloric value nor C-F properties. For health purposes, light dressings of seasoned vinegar and sugar with only a few drops of oil are best. One can buy imitation mayonnaise with only half to two-thirds the calories of regular mayonnaise (which contains 100 per tablespoon) and with reduced C-F properties. Usually made of hydrogenated soybean oil and starch, it has a consistency and flavor near enough to genuine mayonnaise to warrant its use. Or you can try a low-calorie, low C-F mayonnaise that is easy to make at home if you have a blender or food processor (see recipe on page 158). In view of the advantages of these alternatives, most people should be willing to adjust their taste buds for a reasonable shot at longevity.

We must come to grips with the dairy-products issue. The virtues of butter, cream, and cheese have been sacred since antiquity. In the past, to speak out against them has been considered profane by most, particularly the dairy industry. These people have a point; these foods are loaded with nutrients and essential amino acids. Alas, they are also loaded with C-F lipids. The issue revolves around the hypothesis that it is better to find our essentials in some other foods with less tendency to generate atherosclerosis. This seems sensible enough, except that nothing imparts the flavor that butter and cream do, simply nothing. Again we turn, this time half-heartedly, to the substitutes.

Imitation or whipped margarine does the best job of replacing butter. A base of unsaturated vegetable oils cleverly combined with protein complexes has the appearance and consistency of a rather creamy butter, and as a spread it works quite well. However, in cooking, its deficiencies are obvious. Again, we must bully our taste buds into a compromise.

Recently a product called Butter Buds has been placed on the market. It contains 1 percent of the cholesterol and 6 percent of the calories of the same weight of butter. It is a white powder that dissolves in water to produce a butterlike taste, or it may be sprinkled directly on moist hot foods such as cooked vegetables to achieve the same effect. It is said to be made from butter oil excluding nearly all the fat and calories. Few would claim that its flavor is the same as that of butter, but I have used it extensively as a butter flavor and find it satisfactory.

It is sad to contemplate the loss of all those splendid dishes whose depth of flavor depends so much on the use of butter and cream in their preparation, but intelligence and the love for life will eventually prevail; I predict that a day will come when there will be little or no market for dairy products. I fear that it will not be in our time.

Cheeses are nature's very special combinations of proteins and fat put together by a variety of molds. Cheeses offer us a choice, at least. Most of them—and, I confess, the best—contain so much fat that they are impractical in a sensible diet. A few—cottage cheese, farmer cheese, sapsago, mozzarella, and provolone—are largely protein, and they contain a number of essential amino acids. Regrettably, all of them, with the exception of sapsago, are fairly high in calories. Look for skim-milk cheeses whenever possible for the best chance of finding a lower-calorie food.

Next we come to the great egg controversy. Eggs have served as the ubiquitous substitute for meat since the domestication of the hen. Whenever there has been a lack of meat or time, the willing egg has been pressed into service. It is almost the perfect food, except for one failing: its yolk is chock-a-block with cholesterol, although the white of the egg is innocent of fat. What a pity! The egg is so easy to have around, so easy to prepare in so many different ways, so good to eat. "The incredible, edible egg!" Here, again, there are substitutes, but nutritional chemists are no match for the hen. Imitation eggs scramble quite nicely, especially if one supplements their flavor with a little chopped onion, meat, or cheese. The mixture can be used in cooking, too, but with indifferent success. It is low in cholesterol, but its calorie count is approximately the same as the real McCoy. All of this brings us to another compromise. Most authorities agree that two eggs a week, used in whatever manner we care to prepare them, supply us with valuable nutrient essentials without jeopardizing our C-F intake.

Our chief sources of proteins are meats. For the sake of simplicity, we include poultry and fish. America is the greatest meat-eating country in the world; beef and pork surpass all other varieties by a wide margin. Meat is muscle, and all muscle contains some fat, fat that cannot be cut away because it is embedded around the muscle fibers. Pork contains more fat than beef, and beef more than any other meat. When the fat accumulates to the degree that it is visible to the naked eye, it is called marbling. Remember that flavor is borne by the lipids in most foods. It is the infiltrating fat that imparts the wonderful taste to good beef. Infiltrated fat also makes the meat tender. Before they are sent to market, cattle and hogs are penned up in close quarters to restrict their movement and consequently their muscles. They are then fed a diet high in calories which they convert into fat. The best beef—the most flavorful, the most tender, and the most expensive—is more than half fat, although some of this fat can be cut away. An ounce of suet contains about 250 calories; a single drop that drips from your broiler is worth around five. Marbled fat is reduced by broiling, but, however it is prepared, each ounce of beef contains about 100 calories, a moderate serving about 300 calories, and a man-sized half-pound about 800. If it is good beef it is also laden with C-F lipids. Clearly, whoever orders a steak or roast beef dinner under the illusion that it is the best way to eat a low-calorie, low-cholesterol meal is indulging in fantasy. Beef contains many of the essential amino acids; what a pity that they come at such an exhorbitant cost in terms of health and longevity!

Fowl and fish are good and dependable sources of protein. Chicken farming was once a last-resort occupation for people who had failed at more glamorous ways of making a living. Apparently, the people who went into it no longer need our concern. In the past thirty-five years, those who have produced chickens for the market have changed American eating standards. Chicken used to be the dish we had on Sunday. Today it is the dish to fill the hiatus when we don't have beef, lamb, or pork. Chicken has become the poor man's solace and substitute for the more expensive meats. The overworked chicken has done a commendable job. Its praiseworthy career has apparently just begun.

The white meat of chicken has about a third of the calories of a good piece of beef and little more than half as much C-F lipid. It lends itself to literally dozens of ways of preparation, many with an only minimally traumatic effect upon our aortas. Chicken is the hope of the hungry human, and it is still affordable. Lest we become carried away by these accolades, there are some precautions.

Chicken (and all other poultry) fried or roasted, has a cozy image, covered with savory brown skin pocked with feather follicles, cherished images associated with Thanksgiving and Christmas holidays. We have also learned to like the flavor of roasted chicken skin—fat, feather follicles, and all. When a chicken is properly dressed, most of the free fat is withdrawn and discarded. But the skin remains, and the skin is where almost all the fat is. When I say that chicken has only about a third of the calories of beef, I am speaking of a skinned chicken. The patient, obliging chicken will simply have to create a new image for itself. It will look a bit naked at first without its skin, but perhaps if we remember all those feather follicles the adjustment will be easier.

A few years ago, fish began to rival chicken as a solution for our protein needs. Except in seaport towns, however, it has been losing the contest in recent times. Chicken farming is a man-made industry. It can expand as far as man cares to support it. Fish, alas, are still made by a less controllable authority. Their supply can be exhausted and there is nothing much we can do about it. Have you tried to buy a Maine lobster recently? Or jumbo gulf shrimp? These delectable crustaceans are approaching the end of their trails. There will always be an occasional lobster and, I suppose, an occasional shrimp, because they will have government protection before they are completely extinct; but for most of us, they will be unobtainable, at least for a casual dinner. Already there have been subtle deviations to fill the breach. It is now legal to bill South African lobster as "lobster tail" on the menu. In a way it is the tail of one kind of lobster, but if you thought that you were getting Maine lobster when you ordered lobster tails you were almost certainly being hoodwinked. Many people don't make the distinction; those of us who have eaten the genuine article and know that there is no substitute feel cheated.

There are still lots of fish in the ocean, and from a medical standpoint fish is the best source of a low–C-F lipid, low-caloric protein of the highest quality. Fortunately, fish usually withstands freezing somewhat better than beef or lamb. Fish can be prepared as easily as chicken, although there aren't as many variations to relieve monotony. And we must remember not to drown our seafood in butter as a consolation.

Some people, troubled with a weight problem, feel sanctimonious when they restrict themselves to an occasional vegetable dinner. Secure in their belief that all vegetables are low in calories, they fill their plates with extra large helpings of four or even five vegetables. This is one reason why they have a weight problem. They should remember that horses, cattle, and even elephants are completely herbivorous. Vegetable does not automatically mean low calorie. It is true that some vegetables contain relatively few calories—celery, spinach, asparagus, lettuce, cucumbers, and mushrooms among them. One can prepare a delectable meal with braised mushrooms, celery cooked in chicken stock, and asparagus with a light béchamel sauce.

Most vegetables should be blanched as soon as possible after picking. This is because the cells of all vegetables contain enzymes that continue to function after the vegetable has been picked. These enzymes change the simpler carbohydrates to starch, which alters the flavor. Heat destroys the enzymes, thereby stopping the conversion to starch. Sweet corn, contrary to popular belief, can be kept two or three days if it has been blanched immediately after picking. The New England admonition, "Put on the kettle before going out to pull the corn," still holds, but dinner may be delayed for days without substantially altering the flavor of this great vegetable if it is blanched in advance. Leaving blanched vegetables in water ensures that they will not dry out and toughen. All green vegetables, especially string beans, should be blanched the moment they reach the kitchen.

How best to perform this important routine? The water volume must be large, about ten times that of the vegetables, and it should be boiling furiously when the vegetables are dropped in. The large volume is necessary to prevent the water's cooling when the vegetables are added, which defeats the purpose of the operation. Blanching time varies with the vegetable. Asparagus takes five minutes, string beans seven, for example. Consult any good general cookbook for specifics. After blanching, rinse the vegetable in cold water.

It is widely held that boiling vegetables in a large amount of water and then draining the cooking water down the sink is the height of culinary folly. Cooks shake their heads and warn us that we are throwing away all the minerals and vitamins. They should know that most minerals cannot be boiled out of vegetable cells and most of the soluble vitamins have already been destroyed by the heat. Moreover, these substances can be replaced by a pill in the morning. Blanching vegetables is just about as important as pasteurizing milk. In a way the processes are analogous: pasteurization inactivates bacteria, blanching inactivates destructive enzymes.

Dried beans of all varieties and dried peas are the best vegetable sources of protein, but they are high in calories. Fresh beans or peas supply about 25 calories per ounce, or fewer than 100 calories for a generous serving. Baked beans and split peas provide approximately three times that number.

Most fruits have little or no fat and a reasonably small number of calories. Cantaloupe is a worthy example; avocado the most notable exception. In Mexico the avocado is called "peasants' butter." It has about 100 calories per ounce, practically all of which is fat. For those who are trying to reduce, the delicious and intriguing avocado must go.

One thing more should be said before closing this chapter. There is at present a fad concerned with what is generally known as "natural food." Natural food is presumably anything that can be eaten that has not been altered from its natural state. I suppose the idea arises in the knowledge that man is the only species that alters the chemistry of his food before ingesting it. Animals eat food as nature produces it and thrive; ergo: so should we. The concept is valid as long as it does not conflict with the findings of our modern nutrition scientists. Most prepared foods are superior, in one or another specific way, in nutritional value to those that occur naturally. The food faddist should probably depend on the trained personnel of the Pure Food and Drug Administration and our physiologists, our metabolists, our chemists, to tell him which prepared foods should be omitted from his diet and those that science has proven superior to the crude natural products.

14

Planning for Weight Reduction

Most Americans are too fat!

Nature intended a life of chronic hunger, the weaker of us to die of starvation. This blunt statement expressed in a more scientific, if perhaps not kinder, way is the doctrine of survival of the fittest. Sing if you like of the beauties and the bounties of nature, but kindness and mercy she knows not of. She looks tolerantly on the male as long as he has the potential for insemination; she pampers the female as long as she will assume the burdens of childbearing. These missions accomplished, their agents are abandoned with brute callousness. Even our teeth give way to the ravages of age. The need of humankind to eat after the period of reproduction has never been nature's concern. She is only interested in the preservation of the species.

For over a million years, man has endeavored to make up for nature's deficiencies, correct her inequities, outwit her brute objectivity. He has invented his own teeth to replace the inadequate ones he was given. He also has seen to it that he has something to use them on, and let the species go hang. But nature has retained the upper hand. Fat people do not live as long as those of normal weight. We know that obesity is associated with atherosclerosis, which in one way or another kills about half of us. Obesity is also implicated in diabetes, some kinds of heart disease, arthritis, gall-bladder disease, and cirrhosis in beer drinkers. You rarely die of obesity per se, but it does keep bad company. The fat man may be a jolly man, but he should be sure his life insurance is paid up.

It is difficult to find unanimity of opinion about what is normal weight. The tables with which most of us are familiar were calculated for life-insurance companies by striking an average of the weights of thousands of people of the same age and height. Because most Americans are heavier than they should be for their own health and longevity, these figures have come to be considered excessively high by most authorities. Taking into account most biological factors, metabolists have since reduced the figures to more realistic levels. You will find moderate variations in a number of tables that are widely used today, but they are based on averages of people who have lived normal life spans. Such a table is given below and a good many people may want to use it. It is your privilege, but I believe you should first understand the implications outlined below.

It is my considered opinion that the figures given above are

TABLE 1:
AVERAGE ADULT WEIGHTS

Height measured without shoes; weight taken without clothes. For light frames subtract five pounds (2.27 kg); for heavy frames add nine pounds (4.08 kg).

MALES

Height	*Weight*
5′ 3″ / 160 cm	121 lbs. / 55 kg
5′ 4″ / 163 cm	127 lbs. / 58 kg
5′ 5″ / 165 cm	132 lbs. / 60 kg
5′ 6″ / 168 cm	137 lbs. / 62 kg
5′ 7″ / 170 cm	140 lbs. / 64 kg
5′ 8″ / 173 cm	144 lbs. / 65 kg
5′ 9″ / 175 cm	151 lbs. / 69 kg
5′ 10″ / 178 cm	154 lbs. / 70 kg
5′ 11″ / 180 cm	160 lbs. / 73 kg
6′ 0″ / 183 cm	163 lbs. / 74 kg
6′ 1″ / 185 cm	171 lbs. / 78 kg
6′ 2″ / 188 cm	174 lbs. / 79 kg
6′ 3″ / 191 cm	179 lbs. / 81 kg

FEMALES

Height	Weight
5′ 0″ / 152 cm	100 lbs. / 45 kg
5′ 1″ / 155 cm	102 lbs. / 46 kg
5′ 2″ / 158 cm	105 lbs. / 48 kg
5′ 3″ / 160 cm	109 lbs. / 49 kg
5′ 4″ / 163 cm	116 lbs. / 53 kg
5′ 5″ / 165 cm	119 lbs. / 54 kg
5′ 6″ / 168 cm	123 lbs. / 56 kg
5′ 7″ / 170 cm	127 lbs. / 58 kg
5′ 8″ / 173 cm	132 lbs. / 60 kg
5′ 9″ / 175 cm	137 lbs. / 62 kg
5′ 10″ / 178 cm	142 lbs. / 64 kg
5′ 11″ / 180 cm	147 lbs. / 67 kg
6′ 0″ / 183 cm	151 lbs. / 69 kg

still too high. A normal life span is only one of the factors that should be considered in setting up such a table. If excess weight is associated with atherosclerosis, and I believe it to be at least a factor, then the best possible weight would be the average of those people *without* atherosclerosis. Such figures are not available now and will not be until we have conquered atherosclerosis at least to the extent that large numbers of people who do not suffer from it are available for analysis.

I have spent an active lifetime evaluating the association of atherosclerosis, body weight, and longevity. Twenty years ago I constructed a table of what appeared to me to be the best possible weights of adult men and women. As I have applied these figures over the years I have encountered no sound reason for changing them. I am aware that these weights are low by the standards of most authorities, but I have observed many people who have maintained them and have remained healthy and exceedingly active. It is my conviction that these people will live longer than those who maintain weights from five to fifteen pounds heavier and that they will ultimately reveal less atherosclerosis. It is the latter premise that seems to me to be most important, too important to dismiss simply because achieving and maintaining these weights demand a greater amount of self-discipline.

Table 2: Modified Adult Weight Table

Height measured without shoes; weight taken without clothes. For light frames subtract five pounds (2.27 kg); for heavy frames add nine pounds (4.08 kg).

MALES

Height	Weight
5′ 3″ / 160 cm	120 lbs. / 54 kg
5′ 4″ / 163 cm	123 lbs. / 56 kg
5′ 5″ / 165 cm	126 lbs. / 57 kg
5′ 6″ / 168 cm	129 lbs. / 59 kg
5′ 7″ / 170 cm	132 lbs. / 60 kg
5′ 8″ / 173 cm	136 lbs. / 62 kg
5′ 9″ / 175 cm	139 lbs. / 63 kg
5′ 10″ / 178 cm	142 lbs. / 64 kg
5′ 11″ / 180 cm	146 lbs. / 66 kg
6′ 0″ / 183 cm	150 lbs. / 68 kg
6′ 1″ / 185 cm	154 lbs. / 70 kg
6′ 2″ / 188 cm	158 lbs. / 72 kg
6′ 3″ / 191 cm	161 lbs. / 73 kg

FEMALES

Height	Weight
5′ 0″ / 154 cm	101 lbs. / 46 kg
5′ 1″ / 155 cm	104 lbs. / 47 kg
5′ 2″ / 157 cm	107 lbs. / 49 kg
5′ 3″ / 160 cm	110 lbs. / 50 kg
5′ 4″ / 163 cm	113 lbs. / 51 kg
5′ 5″ / 165 cm	116 lbs. / 53 kg
5′ 6″ / 168 cm	120 lbs. / 54 kg
5′ 7″ / 170 cm	124 lbs. / 56 kg
5′ 8″ / 173 cm	128 lbs. / 58 kg
5′ 9″ / 175 cm	132 lbs. / 60 kg
5′ 10″ / 178 cm	136 lbs. / 62 kg
5′ 11″ / 180 cm	140 lbs. / 64 kg
6′ 0″ / 183 cm	144 lbs. / 65 kg

If we calculate the weight of a thousand young athletes and compare it with that of a thousand sedentary men in their forties, a surprising disparity will become apparent. The younger men are what nature defines as her healthiest specimens; that is, they are the best fitted for the physical vicissitudes of life and they are from five to ten pounds lighter than their elders even though they have more muscle. My table is only an approximation; you may add or subtract three to five pounds if you like, but you would do well to plan your dietary intake to achieve the weights given here rather than those of more orthodox tables.

These low weight figures may startle and disturb you. They should not. A nationally known cardiologist contended that we should strive to maintain throughout the remainder of our lives the weight we had when we were twenty-five. I believe that this is good advice. Like most good advice it is not easy to follow. But it is realistic and it pays big dividends if you are properly motivated.

At the outset, if you want to lose weight you should establish the fact that you are too heavy for your best health. Then you should make a serious attempt to find out why. It is true that a rare case of exaggerated obesity is caused by a disturbance in the fundamental metabolic processes—an abnormality of food utilization for one or more types of nutrients. We usually classify these under four separate headings.

Endocrine factors: Dysfunction of one or more of the endocrine glands is a rare cause of obesity, but if other causes cannot be identified, this must be investigated before it can be ruled out. In rare cases, an underfunctioning thyroid gland is at fault. Overfunction of the adrenal glands or certain cells in the pancreas may lead to localized fat deposits. Atrophy of the ovaries, characterized by shrinking and decreased secretion, encourages obesity after menopause.

Brain lesions: Rare lesions such as tumors arising within some areas of the brain (usually in the pituitary gland or hypothalamus), contribute to obesity by eliminating the sense of satiety. These lesions are usually *accompanied* by other signs and symptoms more dramatic than weight gain.

Metabolic factors: There are no data to support the commonly held belief that absorption of food is more efficient in the obese. Recently there has been a report based on experimental work that suggested that the cells of some obese patients contain enzymes that metabolize nutrients to form fat more efficiently than normal. Certain alterations in the metabolism of insulin, whose deficient production is the usual cause of diabetes, are associated with obesity. What actually goes wrong is not fully understood, but it is clear that this is a rare occurrence. People who are overweight should have their urine checked for sugar.

Decreased energy expenditure: Every movement that you make must be provided with the expenditure of calories, the number depending on the amount of exercise. It is possible to have a less-than-average caloric intake and still gain weight by leading a completely sedentary life.

If these four causes for excessive weight can reasonably be ruled out, then you are like most everyone else: eating too much because you are undisciplined. If you want to maintain your present weight, calculate the number of calories needed by consulting the following table.

TABLE 3:
DAILY ADULT CALORIC NEEDS

Height measured without shoes. For a small frame subtract 120 calories; for a large frame add 150.

MALES

Height	*Calories*
5′ 3″ / 160 cm	2,021 cal.
5′ 4″ / 163 cm	2,070
5′ 5″ / 165 cm	2,130
5′ 6″ / 168 cm	2,175
5′ 7″ / 170 cm	2,235
5′ 8″ / 173 cm	2,310
5′ 9″ / 175 cm	2,370
5′ 10″ / 178 cm	2,430
5′ 11″ / 180 cm	2,490
6′ 0″ / 183 cm	2,565
6′ 1″ / 185 cm	2,640
6′ 2″ / 188 cm	2,730
6′ 3″ / 191 cm	2,805

FEMALES

Height	*Calories*
5′ 0″ / 152 cm	1,700 cal.
5′ 1″ / 155 cm	1,725
5′ 2″ / 157 cm	1,770
5′ 3″ / 160 cm	1,800
5′ 4″ / 163 cm	1,845
5′ 5″ / 165 cm	1,875
5′ 6″ / 168 cm	1,950
5′ 7″ / 170 cm	1,995
5′ 8″ / 173 cm	2,040
5′ 9″ / 175 cm	2,130
5′ 10″ / 178 cm	2,175
5′ 11″ / 180 cm	2,235
6′ 0″ / 183 cm	2,295

Let us suppose that you have determined what your weight should be, that you weigh so many pounds in excess of the optimum, and that this overweight is caused by eating more than you need, more than is good for you. Begin by calculating the number of calories needed to maintain your proper weight. You must decrease that number by about 3,500 calories for every pound of fat that you want to lose.

If you intend to lose one pound every four days (which is probably fast enough), subtract about 900 calories from your daily maintenance allotment. Thus if your maintenance intake is 2,100 calories and you intend to lose weight at the rate of one pound every four days, you must reduce your daily intake to 1,200 calories. This may leave you a bit hungry but in good health and with plenty of vigor to carry on your normal routines. If you want to hasten the weight loss or if you prefer exercise to diet restriction, you can calculate the amount of energy expenditure required (one hour of tennis, two hours of walking, one half hour of jogging, etc.) using the table in Chapter 15.

Water weighs one gram per cubic centimeter, about one pound a pint. Water is easy to add to or remove from body tissues; you can sweat away a quart on a very hot afternoon on the tennis court and replenish it all that evening if you drink beer. Fluctuations in the readings of your scale may not reflect an accurate, sensitive figure for your tissue weight. Counter these variations by weighing yourself at the same time each day and disregard unexpected isolated variations of up to two pounds. You can reduce your weight by a couple of pounds in a day or two with a diuretic, but it won't do anything for either your metabolism or your figure.

Before you decide on the method you want to use to reduce your weight, there are a few things that you should know. The most important is that a balanced diet is essential to maintain health. That fact has been challenged dozens of times by imaginative people who are looking for an easier way (and incidentally the money they can extract by exploiting it). There are easier methods than caloric restriction and some of them work, but all of them, as far as I know, are apt to jeopardize your health. The inane suggestion of a pure fat diet has been advertised. It does not merit comment. Pure carbohydrate diets should not be undertaken, even if you could find a shred of validity for doing so. Pure protein diets, seemingly more sensible at first blush, have been reported to cause severe health impairment and even death.

Some people are afraid to stop smoking for fear of gaining weight. There are two fallacies in this hypothesis. First, the smoking habit has little if anything to do with the metabolism of food. The weight-gain threat is a state of mind—if you are convinced that you will gain weight when you stop smoking, you probably will. If you can muster a minimum of self-discipline you need not give it a thought, because there is no physiological relationship between tobacco and food. Second, the smoking habit is perhaps an even greater threat to your longevity than obesity.

A number of drugs have been advocated to promote weight loss. You are well advised to avoid them. None is wholly and satisfactorily effective, and most are frankly injurious to health. They fall into three broad classes.

Purgatives: Although they have been extensively used in the past, the attendant discomforts and health hazards have proven them inadvisable. Vegetable oils for salads and even frying may be cut by a quarter by heavy mineral oil, not for its laxative effect but because mineral oil is not absorbed and so has neither calories nor atherogenic propensity. These mixtures must be tested for taste and tolerance before judging them practical. In these small quantities the chance is negligible that the mineral oil will deplete the body's supply of the oil-soluble vitamins A and D, and most gastrointestinal tracts should be immune from laxative effects.

Endocrine preparations: Avoid them like the plague! None of them is eventually satisfactory, some of them are cumulative and habit forming, all of them are hazardous.

Appetite depressants: Some of these may work—for a time at least—but most of them have bad side effects (emotional instability, sleeplessness, and hypertension), and the patient for whom they are helpful comes to depend on them. When he quits the drug, which he eventually must do, his weight gain is inevitable and usually catastrophic.

There is no easy road to weight reduction via drugs.

Gross obesity has been treated surgically in two ways. Surgeons have actually removed excess abdominal fat by the bucketful. Operative complications are numerous, the chance of bad after-effect is great, and the mortality rate makes the procedure unjustifiable in every case with which I am familiar. A second surgical approach is an intestinal shunt, which inactivates a portion of the small bowel in order to reduce absorption of food. The operative mortality has been figured at 5 percent, the rate of complications at 40 percent. Intestinal function after this procedure is often so deranged that the "cure" is worse than the disease.

Exercise machines have no specific therapeutic advantages. They reduce weight only in proportion to the number of calories expended in their usage. So does jogging; so does walking upstairs. Exercise, when sensibly chosen and indulged in (and when there is no medical reason against it), is very important—in fact, essential—not as much for keeping weight down as for maintaining muscles (including those of the heart) in tone. Remember that nature abhors a functionless part. Disuse precipitates loss of vitality. Exercise machines are a boon to those who are confined to a limited area; to others they are a waste of money.

Consideration of all the weight-reduction advice, nostrums, and machines usually leads to the conclusion that the only reliable and safe reducing method is the limitation of caloric intake. Before embarking on this undertaking, you should understand a little about the physiology involved.

When the chips are down in the struggle to maintain a healthy diet that will ensure normal weight and free us from the dangers of atherosclerosis, we must conclude that fat is the unmitigating offender, everyone's treacherous enemy. It spells double trouble. First of all, a gram of fat yields twice as many calories (9.2) as a gram of carbohydrate or protein. And what isn't burned is stored, at the expense of the figure. The second evil related to fats is that they provide the constituents that go into the making of cholesterol, the offending substance in the plaques of atherosclerosis.

Yes, fat is the real villain, and it is practically ubiquitous. It is a sly and vicious rascal, too. Most of what we call flavors and scents are borne in the essential oils which are a variety of fats, exotic combinations of fatty acids. When the fats are completely extracted, food is left without its differential flavor: it can be only sweet, sour, bitter, or salty. Nature bumbled there, too. To make the living organism want to provide itself with nourishment, she concealed the lure in the least valuable of all the food constituents. She encouraged adequate feeding—and atherosclerosis.

Man has been smart enough to invent the computer and to find his way to the moon. He has been smart but not sagacious. He has not been wise enough to change his tastes to something other than the flavorful fats. Selfishly he has approached the problem from the other side; he has invented imitation bacon, imitation butter, even imitation eggs. Our pigs must be immensely relieved, our cows chagrined, and our hens utterly astonished.

15

The Energy Equation

Calories ingested − energy expended = energy stored as fat.

You don't need a physicist to explain that equation. When we eat more food than we need, we convert the calories that we do not use to supply us energy into neutral fat and store it as blubber. When we want to reduce this excess, we must take in fewer calories than we expend so that our tissues will be obliged to burn stored fat.

Energy balance! It is a deceptively simple formula for what is actually a very complicated matter. We must use up the calories that we ingest or they will have to be stored somewhere, either in the usual storage depots—the belly wall, the buttocks, etc.—or combined with proteins and deposited in more vital locations such as the arterial walls. Normally the stored fats are used the next time there is a call for energy that has not been supplied by such readily available sources as ingested carbohydrates. When unchallenged by this need, these neutral fats accumulate. Other lipids, particularly cholesterol, are linked with proteins. It appears to be the duty of some of these proteins, the high-density lipoproteins (HDLs), to transport cholesterol to the liver, where it is excreted harmlessly in bile. But another type of protein-lipid compound, low-density lipoprotein (LDL), seems to have been designed to carry cholesterol into the cells. If there is a surfeit of cholesterol there, the cells refuse to accept it and turn it back into the blood stream. Where else can it go? It floats about in the blood until a place is found to dump it. Like trash in the streets, it litters the blood passageways. Eventually it is deposited as cholesterol plaques within the blood-vessel walls. Atherosclerosis is on its way.

An increase in stored fats (a polite way of referring to obesity) also promotes atherosclerosis. When needed energy has to come from neutral fats, reconstituted lipid-breakdown products (including cholesterol) are increased. The trouble arises because we have defied one of nature's principles: when population density exceeds food supply, it is the former that must give; death by starvation is the intended result. But man has outsmarted nature by providing a bounty for all that need and an excess for those that are successful. In retaliation, nature strikes back, bringing atherosclerosis with its attendant evils of coronary occlusion, stroke, and peripheral vascular disease.

Energy balance is a complicated matter, but one you must master if you are to survive the strictures of the biological system. You must adjust your energy intake and your energy expenditure until they are approximately equal.

For purposes of this discussion, we may say that part of our energy is used in the process of living while at rest (this is measured as the basal metabolic rate) and the remainder is used in exercise. Every movement we make utilizes at least some energy and thus burns some calories. Exercise is the great variable. The amount of exercise is important in determining the caloric intake necessary to maintain body weight. Some people hoard their energy as misers do their money. They arise in the morning and ride to their offices, sit at their jobs, ride back to their homes, sit through the evening watching television or reading, and then retire to their beds. They spend only a few calories more than that required for basal metabolism. Others may use a great deal more energy even though they, too, may do desk work. They spend much of their day on their feet, standing, walking, climbing stairs. There is a difference, although not as great as we might like it to be, in the caloric expenditure of these two people. Food intake must obviously be adjusted to the caloric need. Because we can voluntarily adjust our caloric expenditure through physical activity, exercise is one means to achieve balance, although not one that is as important as exercise buffs would like to believe.

The following table shows the number of calories required for several types of activity. The numbers represent the caloric expenditure for one hour for each pound of body weight. If you

TABLE 4:
EXERCISE-CALORIE CHART

Activity	*Caloric Expenditure*
Sleeping	0.1
Sitting	0.2
Standing	0.5
Golf (with cart)	1.0
Walking (leisurely)	1.5
Housework	1.5
Bicycling (leisurely)	1.5
Bowling	1.5
Walking (4 miles/hr.)	2.0
Dancing (sedately)	2.0
Golf (no cart)	2.0
Canoeing	2.0
Horseback riding	2.0
Ping-Pong	2.5
Exercising (moderately)	2.5
Tennis	3.0
Bicycling (energetically)	3.5
Volleyball	3.5
Jogging	4.0
Swimming	4.0
Skating	4.0
Skiing	4.0
Dancing (all out)	4.5
Handball	4.5
Running	5.5
Rowing	5.5
Basketball	6.5
Climbing stairs	7.0

want to know how many calories you are using during a given exercise, multiply the number in the chart by the number of hours that you spend and multiply that by your weight in pounds. The items on the chart have been arranged from the mildest exercise, such as golf with a cart or walking leisurely, to the most demanding, such as basketball or climbing stairs.

Thus, if you take a leisurely walk for about an hour over a level course and you weigh 150 pounds, you will probably expend about 1.5 calories per pound of body weight, a total of 225 calories. If you just sat still during that time, you would have spent 30 calories, so you used only about 195 more by exercising.

It has always taken a lot of hard work to compensate for indiscretion. Some people are so lazy they burn as little as 1,700 calories per day. These people make fat of all calories in excess of that amount.

If you study the exercise-calorie table, you will note that even sleeping requires the expenditure of some energy, the basal metabolic rate used in contraction of heart muscle and in maintaining body heat. The greatest amount of energy is required to lift a given weight from one level to a higher one. This is most commonly experienced lifting one's own body, that is, when one climbs stairs. You will note that this exercise is the most energy-consuming on the chart.

Remember that overexercise is hazardous. Respiratory distress is a sign that the exercise is probably too arduous. "Bone tiredness" is another good indication that the would-be athlete has overextended him or herself. Anyone over fifty-five who encounters real fatigue (you are usually amply aware of its occurrence) should eschew pride and go to bed until the feeling has passed.

In view of the jogging fad that has swept the country, there is a good deal you should know about it before you undertake a running program. I have been a jogger and I believe that those who are fit and who enjoy jogging reap certain benefits from the practice, although not as much as some ebullient accounts would have us believe. Moreover, and more important for our discussion, running is not a significant means of losing weight. It is a moderately strenuous form of exercise; it makes definite demands upon the cardiovascular and respiratory systems that can be damaging if those systems are incapable of withstanding the strain. It is furthermore very hard on certain joints, regardless of training and caution in execution. Nature has constructed our weight-bearing joints to provide a limited amount of service. Like some commercially manufactured products, they are designed with a built-in obsolescence—joints wear out just as the shock absorbers on our cars do. When man's life expectancy was forty-five years, his joints served him quite adequately. Now that we can expect to live almost twice that long, we should be provided with an auxiliary set to see us through. Alas, we are not so provided; and most of us will suffer from some degree of osteoarthritis, a degenerative joint disease, during the later years of our lives. Jogging, if it continues to be the popular fad that it is now, will contribute to an increase in incidence and severity of osteoarthritis, especially in the knee and foot joints, and to its onset at an earlier age.

Jogging is not an effective way of losing weight, not even of maintaining a normal weight. The jogger spends approximately 4 calories per pound of body weight per hour of activity. If you weigh 135 pounds and jog for half an hour, you will burn up only about 200 more calories than you would standing still (270 less the 70 you would have burned at routine activity), considerably less than the number of calories contained in the ham-and-cheese sandwich you will probably eat to satisfy the appetite aroused by jogging.

Jogging tones the leg and belly muscles and certainly promotes pulmonary ventilation, at least while on the road. Also, it probably slows the pulse rate, which may be good, although the effect on longevity of a lower pulse rate has not been undisputably determined. A modest body of evidence is emerging to show that those who jog throughout middle age have higher levels of HDL than people of similar age who are sedentary. Their HDL/LDL ratio is also favorable. It is still unproven that a middle-aged person may take up running and thereby increase his HDL level and, presumably, thereby decrease his vulnerability to heart attack.

If you try jogging and hate it, I doubt that it is worth the candle. Despite publicity to the contrary, I do not believe that jogging is for older people. I do not know what the cease-jogging age is and it probably varies widely according to physical state and condition, but if you are over sixty, I suggest you be cautious. There are other contraindications. If there is any evidence of chronic pulmonary disease (emphysema or bronchiectasis), or cardiac insufficiency, whatever its cause (rheumatic scarring, coronary insufficiency, hypertension), or if there is clinical evidence of arthritis of the knees or bad feet (fallen arches), then you should not attempt jogging without an okay from a competent physician. Grossly obese people should not jog. If they can first reduce their weight by dietary control to a level that allows running without excessive exertion, then they may undertake a modified jogging program with profit.

I suggest that anyone contemplating a jogging program read something about it before starting, but I am at a loss for an authoritative source to recommend. Joggers who write on the subject appear to me to be biased; writers who do not jog appear to lack sufficient knowledge.

What is said for jogging goes for planned exercise programs at home or in a gymnasium. Such activities are apt to be too strenuous and end up by discouraging the participant from exercising at all. Competitive sports (tennis, handball) are excellent if you enjoy them; I doubt that they accomplish much if you do not.

These are all exercises that most people would consider arduous. If physical fitness depended on strenuous exercise, we would never have achieved our longevity average of seventy-two years. But physical fitness does depend upon active utilization of all our faculties. Nature abhors a state of disuse. Functional failure of any of our anatomical parts, even for as short a time as a matter of weeks, induces atrophy. Atrophy is a term pathologists use to describe the condition of a tissue or organ that is reduced not only in size but in actual number of cellular constituents. All body tissues are subject to this process. If a patient lies motionless in bed for more than a week or two his muscles begin to shrink in size and strength. Even an unused bone will atrophy. For example, a broken arm is usually x-rayed and put in a cast for a matter of weeks. When the cast is removed, the arm is usually x-rayed again. A comparison will clearly show a diminution of bone density in the later x-ray. Many herbivorous animals have large storage sacks attached to their large intestines. As the digestive system of man evolved over the centuries, this storage area became unnecessary and nonfunctional. Now it exists as a small wormlike appendage, the vermiform appendix. With loss of function, it atrophied.

The opposite of atrophy is hypertrophy. Many of our tissues and organs become larger and capable of greater function if challenged by use. The muscle-builder may enlarge any group of muscles by special exercises. When the work load is increased, the heart, a special kind of muscle, will hypertrophy as long as its blood supply remains great enough to meet the demand. Endocrine glands (thyroid, adrenals, and others) will increase in size and function under excessive and continuous stimulation. Hypertrophy is a built-in reserve designed to meet the demands of stress. To the best of my knowledge, no one has ever proven that cardiac hypertrophy is preferable to the normal state, or that it increases longevity. I know of no statistics to prove that athletes live longer than those who exercise less strenuously but do maintain their anatomical parts in use.

The atrophy of disuse is bad and the hypertrophy of overuse is probably not beneficial. I suggest the middle road is the sensible course. I believe that jogging and other arduous exercises are for most people above the median and unnecessarily severe. I believe that we should maintain activity of all our parts, especially our muscles (including our hearts) and our brains, all of our lives. Dr. Paul White was a world-renowned heart specialist. He insisted that riding his bicycle daily contributed greatly to his longevity. As he lived well into his nineties, I am inclined to agree.

Anyone who thinks about it will probably be able to recall at least one person who had the exercise routine of a three-toed sloth and who lived to be ninety years old. We should always remember that when we construct a curve of incidence there must always be at least one person at each end no matter how many thousands are at the crest. You could probably find a septuagenarian stunt man if you searched hard enough, but his survival would not change the rates for accident insurance among stunt men.

16

Losing Weight

Let us suppose that after a sober consideration of the matter you are willing to forgo certain gustatory pleasures in the reasonable expectation that your life will be prolonged by a decade or more. You decide to reduce. Unless you are in radiant health, it is probably advisable to consult your physician and have a physical examination before you undertake this project. There are some latent diseases, such as diabetes, hypotension, and certain anemias, that should be ruled out before anyone embarks on an unsupervised diet.

Having decided how much you should weigh for health and longevity, how do you achieve this weight without adopting the life of an ascetic? It isn't easy. Nor can it be done effectively and happily simply by limiting the amount of the food you ingest. Quality is an important factor, too; the *kind* of food is as important as the amount, and it almost certainly entails an alteration in your tastes. A moment of truth comes when you face the realization that there are certain foods that you simply must not eat, no matter how much you enjoy them. There go breakfasts of fried eggs and bacon, lunches of avocado salad and apple pie, and dinners of roast pork with ice cream for dessert. Is the banishment of such items as deep-fried meats and vegetables, pastry desserts, nuts, and candy worth another decade or two of life? If you don't think so there is no purpose in reading this book. Put it down now, arrange for a coffin—a sturdy one—and get that jar of peanut butter down from the shelf.

There are those who balk at the discipline entailed, protesting, "Steak is my favorite dish and I have no intention of giving it up in order to achieve a subnormal weight!" In truth, steak is not the great offender for those seemingly unable to lose weight. Rather, it is the victim of misguided intention. It certainly should not be recommended in large amounts for a slenderizing diet, but it is not all that fattening and few of us can afford to eat it often enough to cause serious weight problems. However, if you familiarize yourself with calorie charts and intelligent cooking techniques, you will open up a new culinary world in which eating becomes more pleasant and more interesting than it has ever been before. The French, who have been the leaders in the culinary arts for more than a century, would hasten to agree. A new style of cooking has been initiated by Paul Bocuse, who has written "for the first time cuisine and dieting are no longer contradictions," and Michel Guerard, who originated *cuisine minceur*.

When a sensible diet has been designed and seriously adopted, body weight gradually falls to an optimum level. You look better and feel better. You will probably have had to endure some alterations in your eating habits and, more important, your tastes. It isn't necessarily easy, but it is certainly worth it.

Having decided what system you intend to use, you should provide yourself with one of the legion of the available calorie guides; any will do as long as it lists all foods, particularly packaged foods, with their brand names. These books have the tendency to give calorie values in terms of a variety of measurements: ounces, tablespoonsful, servings, slices, and size in inches; it makes comparisons difficult and calculations vague. Choose a reference that lists all values in ounces.

Then do a bit of homework. Learn the caloric values of the common foods, particularly fats, and memorize a list of high-risk foods such as lard, butter, cream, cheese, nuts, chocolate, and as many others as you feel you will be tempted to use. You should also memorize a list of low-calorie foods such as mushrooms, asparagus, shrimp, green beans, cantaloupe, and flounder. Take your calorie guide with you to the market and use it, use it, use it until calorie values become second nature.

Next, provide yourself with two scales, a reliable bathroom scale and a kitchen scale calibrated in ounces. No need to buy the kind of kitchen scale equipped with a tank for weighing liquids; you will rarely use the tank. It is enough to remember that a pint is a pound and sixteen ounces make either. Keep the scale on the kitchen counter where your meals are prepared. At first you will use it for almost everything you eat. With experience you will find that you will need it less and less. Until your weight has reached the level that you feel it should be, make a fairly accurate estimate of the number of calories of every meal—in fact, of everything you eat.

By consulting the tables in Chapter 14, calculate what your weight should be and the number of pounds you should lose. You should have a rather accurate idea of the activity expended in your daily routine. Count this as baseline activity. Now estimate the caloric requirement for any additional exercise.

In weight reduction it is wise to plan a loss of one pound about every four days. It can be done much more rapidly by fasting, but such attempts usually end in failure because fasting is abnormal and difficult. For each pound to be lost you must reduce your maintenance caloric level by 3,500 calories. If you choose to take four days in the process you should reduce your maintenance level by a fourth the total, or 900 calories each day. For most people this is a reasonable amount and one they can live with. To this number add the calories used in additional exercise.

If you calculate that the maintenance level of your optimum weight is 2,500 calories at routine activity and you want to lose one pound every four days, reduce your daily maintenance intake by 900 to 1,600 calories. Suppose you play tennis for one hour each day. Your optimum weight is 150 pounds and you spend 3 calories for each pound, or 450 calories. Remember that had you been routinely active for that hour instead of playing tennis, you would have burned up at least 150 calories (1 calorie for every pound of your body weight) so you have used only 300 extra calories (450 less 150). You can add these 300 exercise-reduced calories to your reduced maintenance allotment. By using your bathroom scale daily under controlled circumstances, you may be gratified to learn how accurately you can control and calculate your weight reduction.

Some people like to initiate a weight-reduction program with a short period of fasting. This is permissible providing there are no medical factors against it—check with your doctor. If obesity is a serious problem, these short periods (never longer than one week unless under a doctor's supervision) may be practiced as often as once a month. Breakfast should be limited to black, unsweetened coffee. Lunch should consist of a cup of bouillon and two slices of very thinly sliced toast or one regular slice of bread, toasted and split horizontally to make two pieces. These may be spread lightly with imitation margarine. Dinner should be the same as lunch. The total caloric value of this day's food will not exceed 200 calories. Some people like to practice one day of such fasting each week. This allows them a little more dietary freedom during weekends.

Remember that such a fasting diet allows no alcoholic beverages. If you forego the fasting stage or have completed it and you wish to indulge in a cocktail, figure each ounce and a half of liquor (whiskey, gin, or vodka) at 150 calories. And if you choose a mixer other than club soda or water or one of the diet mixes add that to the caloric total.

We know that fats pose a serious threat in the development of atherosclerosis, the great killer of our age. (Cancer is a vicious killer, too, more dramatic and better publicized, but it is responsible for fewer than a third the number killed by the complications of atherosclerosis.) Certain fats are apparently more atherogenic than others. At this writing it appears that the saturated fats are the most culpable. Most of these are of animal origin; lard, butter, and cream are the worst. Pork contains the highest percentage of fat among the commonly used meats; beef is next, then lamb. A considerable portion of the fat in fowl resides in skin. When skinned, the white meat of chicken has about a third the fat of pork. It is the least fat of the four available types of fowl; turkey is next. Duck and goose are too fat for consideration.

Most fish contain less fat than either fowl or meat. The shell fish—scallops, clams, and mussels but excluding shrimps—are particularly low in fats. Such fish as mackerel, sardines, bluefish, and tuna are oily and high in lipids.

By and large, vegetables and fruits contain little or no fat. There are exceptions, notably avocados. All nuts contain large amounts of fat, up to two-thirds their weight although much of this fat is of the unsaturated variety. Cooking oils are extracted from corn, olives, sunflower seeds, peanuts, cotton seeds, and soybeans. The oils from the first three of these are preferred because they are less saturated.

The saturated fats constitute a large and heterogeneous group of lipids, mostly animal in source (though not entirely), of which cholesterol is only one. There is a growing market for foods that taste enough like fat to make them palatable yet whose saturated-fat content is low enough to allow their inclusion in a low-fat diet. There is a mayonnaise that contains about half the fat of ordinary mayonnaise. There are artificial eggs that contain no cholesterol and bacon that has only a vague resemblance to pork. There are at least three brands of a lecithin spray that help prevent sticking while frying. Those who understand the threat of atherosclerosis should explore all these possibilities. Most of them require some getting used to, but if they serve as an ally in the revolt against the great killer, they merit attention and respect.

You may eat as much protein as you like providing it is part of a balanced diet. The so-called protein additives rarely add anything of value and they are risky to use without a physician's supervision. The trouble with ordinary proteins available at the food markets is that in order to be innocuous they should be free of fat. All meats contain some fat, and fat of the wrong type. Many people order a steak and a salad for dinner and feel righteous in so doing. Actually, beefsteak is about half fat (the better quality the steak, the more fat it contains), and the fat is saturated. You can eat the same amount of skinless chicken breast by weight for about a third the calories.

Carbohydrate calories are blameless as long as there are not too many of them. When caloric need is satisfied by carbohydrates the tissues convert the excess into fat and store it in that form. Carbohydrates are a reliable source of immediate energy; in excessive amounts, you might as well eat fats.

The simplest way to design a healthy diet is to reduce the known fats to a minimum. You will still get enough fat to sustain radiant health. A balanced diet requires about 20 percent of the calories to be taken as fats, yet most diets today are about 40 percent fat. If you use ordinary precautions, your lipid intake will almost certainly be in amounts with a wide margin of safety.

You must be aware by now that my real concern is to increase awareness of the incidence and dangers of atherosclerosis. I have noted several times the mortality record of this disease—for it should be considered a disease—and I firmly believe that anything this important deserves our keenest scrutiny and our most earnest consideration. Atherosclerosis is America's most vicious, most ubiquitous enemy! Why have we been so negligent in organizing ourselves against this colossal evil?

We have fallen prey to this disease for two reasons. We eat more than we need, converting the excess energy into fats that foul our blood streams, and we have acquired a taste for foods of high lipid content because fat is where the flavor is. The combination of these two bad habits is probably the most important factor in the acquisition of atherosclerosis. Because we are doing two things that are endangering our health, there should be two things to safeguard it.

We can eat less so that we achieve a balance between our energy intake and our energy expenditure. To do this successfully we must understand that the number of calories that we need for weight maintenance should equal the number used up in exercise. We must be convinced that weight control is more than an esthetic principle; it is a health requirement.

Second, we shall probably have to change our taste preferences. We should understand that man was intended to be herbivorous, that his cells have been programed to metabolize principally polysaccharides, with some protein and only a little fat. It is futile to change our diets when we find no enjoyment in the food we prescribe for ourselves. The choice and preparation of the dishes that are healthful for us, that liberate us from the fear and threat of atherosclerosis, are not easy. We have to be imaginative and willing to spend more time in the kitchen.

Also, we must be willing, in some instances, to pay higher prices for more healthful foods.

The rewards are measured, however, in years. There is no medication, no surgical procedure, no x-ray treatment for atherosclerosis. The treatment is preventive and you are the only one who can administer it. It is a challenge and the most worthwhile endeavor you may ever make.

If you enjoy life, you should understand the basic principles set forth in the preceding chapters. Given supportable reasons for dietary discipline and some suggestions for sidestepping the more unpleasant aspects of healthy diet maintenance, the adoption of a sensible health-promoting diet is really not all that difficult. But don't wait too long to start. Your aorta has no way of warning you that it may be later than you think.

1

A Change in Taste

We seem to be the pawns of nature. Primitive man was helped to survive the perils of his environment by the dictates of his taste buds. His uncle, who rather fancied the taste of decaying flesh, presumedly died of salmonella poisoning before he had a chance to procreate. Others recorded the observation in that strange and wonderful helix that is each man's tablets of Moses. "Thou shalt not" was translated by our taste buds to "Ugh! What a horrid taste. I'd rather starve!"

Now we know that our taste buds have been disloyal. They have carried out their duties, warning us against deleterious foods, through only our reproductive years; then they abandon us to the ravages of atherosclerosis. But modern knowledge is trying to come to our rescue. We know now that we must re-educate our taste buds from early life, teach them to warn us when we are served a chocolate mousse with a whipped-cream topping. "Ugh! What a horrid sight. You'd rather starve."

We can expect nature to rebuke us for our anarchy. "Save your coronaries if you prefer and later feed the crab of cancer." Perhaps, but let us consider the dictates of our taste buds for what they are, a program for sensual pleasure. And that, we should know by now, must be kept in its place.

The true taste sense, which resides in the taste buds on the surface of the tongue, registers only four qualities: sweet, sour, salty, and bitter; but each of these qualities has thousands of nuances when abetted by a competent olfactory sense. The latter probably developed first. In its primitive state, it served as a mechanism to warn of the presence of danger, of an enemy. Then, as the centuries rolled by, the use of the sense of smell was broadened to assist in locating food. It was a natural. If one can smell danger one can extend that proclivity to the association of disagreeable odors with impending injury. With the perception of unpleasant smells came the distinction of pleasant ones and the association of the latter with something good, that is, something to eat. In some mammals, such as many breeds of dog, the ability has become so highly developed that it serves as the animal's most important sense of awareness. In some insects the olfactory sense achieves the proportions of the fantastic. It is said that in some species the presence of a female can be detected by the male for distances of a mile or more through an odor too subtle for the human nose at any range.

Man has played down the alarm function of his olfactory system because his eyes are more efficient at the enemy-detecting aspect of self-preservation. His ears replace his eyes in the dark to alert him to things that go bump in the night. True, we do sniff a piece of meat that may be overhung to make sure it isn't spoiled, but we have lost the ability to identify our enemies by the odor they emit. Perhaps it is just as well, the perfume business being what it is.

We assume that the taste buds, with their rough classification, were an afterthought to protect the undiscriminating glutton from swallowing things that would do him in. "Ugh! Too sour!" A splitting down of this crude division was made possible with the aid of the olfactory sense, out of which the taste sense originated. By combining the two senses, we can classify odors and foods according to the relationship of the molecules of which they are constituted. Because these relationships are almost infinite, the capacity to distinguish variations is almost infinite, especially with education. Without motivation and education, most of us will find a piece of beef thrown from the frying pan onto the plate a fine enough meal. With motivation and education, the same piece of beef must be spread with foie gras and wrapped in a tender crust to appear at table as a Wellington, designed to satisfy the grandest expectations. If you have ever seen a professional wine taster at work, you can appreciate the degree of efficiency to which the senses of smell and taste have been educated along this specific line. Putting a clothespin on a wine taster's nose is like putting a sleight-of-hand artist in a strait jacket.

The quality of a taste can be described only superficially. If you try to make the verbal distinction between the tastes of raspberries and strawberries, the best that you can say is that one is sweeter than the other. If driven further for a distinction, you fall back on "Well, they taste like raspberries."

Whenever we consider changing our tastes we collide head on with an age-old question: are our food tastes indelibly bred into us in the molecular structure of our genes, or are they simply the imprints of family, regional, and racial habit? It is the old debate, nature versus nurture. I am not implying that acquired characteristics can be inherited—certainly not—but the genetic representatives of taste may be chemically bound to genes that under the circumstances promote health and reproduction. If a strong and fertile group becomes genetically conditioned to eating pickled herring, that group will prosper and the demand for herring burgeon. They would continue even after the herring supply were wiped out forever as long as the group maintained its proclivity for reproduction. A taste for herring, although its gene may be located in the same chromosome as that for reproduction, has nothing to do with the matter. Alas, such may be the case for fats, atherosclerosis, and longevity rates. It is what E. O. Wilson calls our "cultural" genetic inheritance.

What matters is that we may have to change some of our dietary tastes if we are to achieve optimum health and better mortality rates. In short, in order to prevent atherosclerosis, we must cut down our fat consumption and regulate our carbohydrate intake to that which we can burn without storage. If it means bucking an inherited preference, I suppose it could present some problems. Whatever its genetic ramifications we must be sure that a change in taste preference will require considerable motivation. We eat the food we do almost certainly because we like it. Likes and dislikes are not easily changed.

Neither are mortality statistics. I remember struggling with the problem on a personal basis. One day at lunch in the hospital, the conversation turned to the relatively new ideas concerning the cause of atherosclerosis. A clinician whose opinions I much admired suggested that we should all drink reconstituted nonfat dry milk. The very thought was repugnant, but I bought some and gave it a try. It didn't taste much like whole milk; in fact, it didn't taste very good at all. I decided that it wasn't for me. Then I happened to read some reports concerning the alarming incidence of atherosclerosis and I remembered Arty, the boy who had been paralyzed by polio and who loved ice cream. That made me go back and read the army report concerning the incidence of coronary occlusion in young draftees stationed in Korea. I made up another batch of powdered milk and this time disliked it less. After two or three weeks it began to taste good. Now I find it difficult to drink any other kind of milk. I actually prefer its taste and consistency to whole milk. It was simply a matter of motivation. I am convinced that proper motivation can change taste, be it genetic or acquired by habit. (I also learned, by the way, that it tastes best when ice cold and if allowed to stand at least an hour after it is mixed and before it is drunk.)

I believe that the entire matter of adopting a modern, healthful diet is based on the necessity of each individual's changing some of his taste preferences from those that are harmful to those that are healthful. I use the term harmful advisedly and in a relative sense. If you are five pounds overweight, just plain peanut butter is harmful; one tablespoon of the best-known brand contains about 100 calories, most of which, if you are overweight, will be stored as fat and some of which will be deposited within the lining of your aorta. I dearly love peanut butter, but I think that for most people, and especially for those who are overweight, it is harmful.

The first step, then, in eating food that is best for us is learning which foods we should acquire a taste for and, even more important, those we must learn to dislike. The Weight Watchers organization discovered this principle years ago and their success is based on it. When you stop to think about it, acquiring a taste must not be too difficult. If you ever used tobacco you had to learn to tolerate a mouthful of choking smoke, a rather remarkable eccentricity, come to think of it. Your first olive and first raw oyster probably didn't taste very good, nor that first sip of strong black coffee without sugar, nor that first spoonful of yogurt. Ripe Camembert cheese, snails, and unborn eels can become delicacies if you put your heart into it. It is not so easy to give up a taste that was once enjoyed—I still swipe a spoonful of peanut butter when no one is looking.

Yes, a taste for most foods can be acquired providing they are not too exotic *and* providing there is a sensible reason and a moderate degree of motivation for doing so. The reason and motivation can scarcely be questioned as long as medical science maintains its belief in the relationship of a fatty diet and atherosclerosis.

If you search out the substitutes for those foods with a high content of saturated fats and make a reasonable attempt to prepare them in a tasteful fashion, it should not be difficult to maintain your intake of fat at a level in the vicinity of 25 percent. Putting the same effort into the search for foods with a high-protein low-fat content should enable you to raise the percentage of protein in your diet without exceeding the lipid tolerance level.

Some metabolists will insist that a balanced diet should consist of about 45 percent fat, an accepted norm over the past century. He who pays little heed to his dietary intake will find that almost 50 percent of everything he eats is fat. The incidence of atherosclerosis being what it is, this can hardly be upheld as an acceptable standard. I suppose that it would be possible to reduce the amount of fat in the diet to a level so low that it is harmful, but I have never encountered or heard of an actual case. The fact is that even if you limit your lipid intake drastically, the percentage will probably not fall far below 25 because of the ubiquitous nature of fat in the foods we eat.

There are two possibly deleterious complications of a high-protein diet. Proteins tend to produce a reduced volume of intestinal waste and thereby change elimination regularity. An intelligent use of low-calorie, high-bulk foods helps to alleviate this complication. So-called natural food stores usually carry a variety of what are labeled "high fiber" foods. These contain a considerable amount of indigestable cellulose, which is supposed to increase the bulk of the intestinal content and aid elimination. It probably serves this purpose but it may also traumatize the delicate linings of the stomach and intestine. If you have any history of peptic ulcer, varicose veins of the esophagus, or hiatal hernia, do not rely on these products because they may cause internal hemorrhage. As for the statistical evidence that high-protein diets make one more likely to develop colon cancer, too little is known of this relationship to make specified recommendations at present.

It is my belief that taste is acquired. Families learn to prefer what is available. Children clamor for food eaten by those they emulate. No one, I feel reasonably sure, would eat *ludefisk* unless conditioned to its taste and smell. Swedes find it palatable because at one time it was the most widely available food in Sweden. When Sweden and Norway were united, the country had an immense coastline and fish was the main source of protein. Winters were long and hard and the dried fish was the best means of avoiding hunger. Now Swedes eat *ludefisk* even when they don't have to because they learned to like it as children. I have always wondered if an infant snatched from his cradle in Sicily and brought up in an igloo north of the Arctic Circle would grow up to prefer pasta to seal blubber. My guess is that he would not. We prefer to eat what we learn to like.

If I were starting a family today, I would do as my pathologist friend did years ago. I would forbid admission to the kitchen of perhaps two dozen food items—see my list of forbidden foods in the next chapter. A glance at this list will disclose what at first appear to be inconsistencies. Salmon, for example, with a fat content of about 70 grams per pound is on the list, and pork, at about 140 grams, is not. But the list was composed with two objectives. All of the items are high in fat content and all can easily be substituted by items that are not. Any of the six oily fishes listed can be replaced by a fish with considerably less fat. Pork is not easy to substitute. All the same, foods like pork, beef, and lamb, which are high in saturated fats but hard to substitute, must be used sparingly, while poultry and the nonoily fish are accentuated.

I believe that if children are not introduced to these foods at home they will grow up without the desire for them. What a blessing never to be compelled to fight the battle against obesity and atherosclerosis! And what a relief not to feel the dread of early coronary disease or terminal senile dementia!

For the rest of us, born and raised by unenlightened parents, the task is not so easy. Life may appear to be a matter of diminishing returns. We were implored to give up cigarettes and most of us over thirty did. We have been warned about the dire consequences of alcoholic indulgence and have risen with heroic purpose to achieve the temperate life. It became necessary for everyone, man, woman, and child, to jog in order to remain fit. Through sleet and snow, drought and drizzle we struggle and strain, puff and pant.

Now it's food! And after that? The "after that" seems to have been doing more than holding its own, judging from the flood of recent literature on the subject. Although many of us find little solace in the philosophy that "butterflies are free," when we contemplate the joys of a bacon-and-peanut-butter sandwich we can probably think of other things that would be more difficult to forego.

That is all it takes to achieve a change in taste.

18

Calories and Coronaries

This is an era of nostrums that attract sick people to Mexico to imbibe an extract of apricot pits, an era of complacent faith that lures the guileless to Quebec in search of miracles, of obesity cures that remove unwanted pounds, an era of natural foods and protein additives, and as many diet books as there are those who can get them published. Which way does the innocent victim, the average citizen, turn? How does he know the proper course by which to salvage his arteries? I suppose that the most effective solution would be for everyone to acquire a medical degree, but that would take from four to fourteen years and would be very, very expensive. The following pages are written to serve as guideposts for the distraught, whose training has not provided them directions through this jungle of mercenary advice.

To begin with, we must all have the conviction that the two greatest threats to physical well-being and longevity are atherosclerosis and obesity. So convinced, we make the initial confession that most of us eat too much and too much of the wrong kinds of foods.

The next step is to make sure that we understand the principles of the mechanism of atherosclerosis and the means by which we hope to avoid it. Atherosclerosis is caused by the gradual and accumulative deposition of cholesterol in the walls of the large and medium-size arteries. It is deposited when it reaches a certain critical level in the blood. There are two possible reasons why it accumulates in abnormal amounts: either the cells that normally metabolize cholesterol are incapable of normal function (congenital hyperlipoproteinemia) or the amount of cholesterol introduced into the blood is too great for the tissue cells to handle. Cholesterol is a lipid, a fatlike substance. It combines with two kinds of protein. In one of these combinations, low-density lipoprotein, cholesterol is carried to the cells in the arterial wall, where it is either accepted for metabolism or refused. In the second type, high-density lipoprotein, cholesterol is carried to the liver, where it is excreted. It should be obvious that when the amount of cholesterol introduced into the blood is greater than the cells can handle, HDL is a beneficial combination, LDL a harmful one. In short, the lower the LDL blood level and the higher the HDL level, the safer we are from the deposition of excess cholesterol and the development of atherosclerosis and its lethal consequences. The cholesterol status can be more simply expressed by measuring all of the cholesterol in the blood and dividing it by the amount of cholesterol in the HDL. This is called the total cholesterol/HDL ratio or CR. The higher the HDL figure, the better the situation, because a higher HDL level results in a more favorable total cholesterol/HDL ratio.

From data that have been gathered up to this time, it appears that a CR of 2.3 is normal for a newborn child, 4.5 for a normal woman, and 5 for a man. It is advisable that we all attempt to keep our CR level at the normal figure or lower if possible. Each of us should have his CR estimated in early childhood to rule out congenital hyperlipoproteinemia, an inborn inability to metabolize cholesterol. The analysis should be repeated in early adult life. If the level is within the normal range, the analysis need not be repeated more often than every ten years until the age of sixty. After that it should probably be made every year. This determination should be made as part of the battery of tests routinely conducted during the annual health maintenance examination, and it should become part of the permanent record your physician maintains for you. There is reasonable evidence today that the CR level may be lowered by means of a diet low in saturated fats. In most people this diet requires a genuine and intense desire for freedom from the consequences of atherosclerosis, coronary disease, stroke, hypertension, and probably senile dementia. No diet can be said to be successful if those following it find it distasteful. Food pleasure is a very strong incentive throughout nature. Clearly, two factors can make the diet successful. The first is the study of the acceptabilities, and the second is the selection from those of the foods that are palatable. These factors are basic to the *nouvelle cuisine* that has become so popular in France and is beginning to find its way on this side of the Atlantic. In the final chapter of this book you will find a number of low-cholesterol, low-calorie menus and, for those that are not obtainable elsewhere, the recipes for the recommended dishes.

Unless certain harmful foods have been prohibited since childhood, we will continue to desire these high-calorie cholesterol formers, which can defeat the program of even the most conscientious dieter. To forestall this failure, I submit a list of twenty-eight common foods that I believe should never be permitted in the kitchen. There are substitutes for all of them, substitutes that make the menu attractive and thereby the diet successful. Of course, this means some alteration in taste preferences for most of us. If that is necessary, it must be attempted.

The worst offenders are the fatty foods that cause both obes-

TABLE 5:
FORBIDDEN FOOD

Lard	Nuts	Sausage
Butter	Coconut	Duck
Margarine	Peanut butter	Goose
Palm oil	Chocolate	Mackerel
Coconut oil	Pastry	Herring
Peanut oil	Cocoa	Salmon
Cream	Mayonnaise	Tuna
Milk (whole)	Bacon	Sardines
Cheese	Frankfurters	Avocados

ity and atherosclerosis, specifically lard, butter, and margarine. For most cooks, putting lard on the forbidden food list means sacrificing pastry, because few pastry cooks will bake without it. Good! Pastries are insidious villains anyway. The substitute for these three saturated fats is imitation margarine, which has a three-to-one ratio of unsaturated to saturated fats and contains about half the calories of butter or lard. If you have had reservations concerning its taste and therefore its use, you will probably be surprised at how quickly these reservations vanish when it is used as a spread.

Most of the fat used in cooking should come from the liquid oils that are available commercially. Of these, four that should be avoided are those made from palm nuts, coconuts, peanuts, and cottonseed. They are the more saturated. Oils from soybeans, corn, and safflower are preferable. Olive oil is somewhere between and those who cherish its flavor in sauces and dressings should use it sparingly.

Next come the dairy products. The members of a generation that has been taught that the healthiest foods in the world are good rich milk, cream, butter, and cheese are apt to go into a state of shock upon hearing that these items are forbidden on the basis of health. The initial reaction is one of indignant rage. Innocent babies of all the mammalian species from hamsters to hominids have been nourished on milk. Whence comes this outrageous blasphemy?

Milk fat, for most, is among the most digestible of lipids. For those in whom the accumulation of atheromatous plaques has not yet begun, it is quite innocent of deleterious effects. The cholesterol ratio of newborn infants is around 2.3, a figure that is exceeded soon after the ingestion of milk fat has begun. This figure is never again attained, except on the most rigid of low-fat diets. By the time the child is two or three years old, yellow streaks may be found in the linings of the aorta. It is believed by most that these deposits are the beginnings of atheromatous plaques.

Some cheeses are relatively fat-free. These should be chosen over those made from cream. But all cheeses have a rich component of casein and casein is one of the accomplices indicted by certain atherogenic research studies. That puts cheese of all kinds among the forbidden foods. The best plan is to rely on skimmed or fat-free milk as a substitute for whole milk. The dried fat-free product is innocent and, after a bit of taste reeducation, acceptable to the taste buds. Many people, I for one, prefer it to fresh nonfat milk, and it is easier to store.

All nuts are rich in lipids and, therefore, high in calories. Nuts are among the most concentrated sources of fattening foods. The delectable nuts, all of them, are best avoided. The peanut is exonerated neither by its humble social status nor by its membership in the legume family.

Chocolate and cocoa are two food products that have little dietary value unless one happens to be scaling mountain peaks or running long distances. The rest of us should eschew them.

Mayonnaise is a problem that deserves special attention. Both rich in egg yolks and high in calories, it is a serious enemy in our war on atherosclerosis and obesity. Nonetheless, deleting it from the diet leaves a significant void. A low-calorie, low-fat dressing that rivals its flavor can be made from a recipe on page 158.

All pork and pork products should be suspect. When broiled, however, well-trimmed pork and ham may be allowed occasionally on the dining table. But bacon and most sausages cannot be rendered (no pun intended) sufficiently low in saturated fat to make them usable. Because frankfurters are usually made of the fatty trimmings of pork and beef, they should rarely be used.

It is regrettable that the selection among poultry is so limited. Of the four types available on the market, only chicken and turkey (with skin removed) can be considered; ducks and geese are excessively fat. As in pork, the fat not only accumulates as masses of blubber that can be cut away, but it infiltrates the muscle bundles in a form that cannot be satisfactorily removed.

The edible fish vary greatly in their fat content. Because there are many varieties with scarcely any lipid, there seems little sense in buying the oily ones. Such fish as flounder, haddock, cod, and red snapper are low in fat and should be used as often as the palate and the purse will permit. When canned salmon and tuna are packed in water they are more acceptable than when packed in oil.

In Mexico, the avocado grows everywhere and its trees are prolific. For the poor Mexican who rarely tastes butter or pork, the avocado is a God-given essential. The North American who needs vegetables and fruits to balance his animal-fat intake should regard the lipid-laden avocado an anathema.

Having determined the kind of food you are going to live on, you must determine the proper amount that will promote optimum health. Each of you must make your own calculations, and having made them, must live by them. A careful reading of Chapters 14, 15, and 16 should help you establish the exact number of calories that will maintain health and vigor.

First decide what you should or want to weigh. Next decide the amount of time you want to spend losing the pounds in excess of your goal. Be aware that most failures are rooted in an attempt to lose weight too fast. If your diet is too austere you are constantly hungry and may feel weak and tired most of the time. Losing weight under these circumstances is a bore, but if you are willing to settle for a gradual loss of approximately four pounds per week and make the effort to provide interesting and tasty foods to achieve this end, it need not be a trial. Following is a list of foods that should be used as often as they are considered palatable. For example, mushrooms and asparagus are two almost perfect reducing foods. They can be prepared in several ways, all of them interesting and delicious, and should be used as often as possible. All the foods listed here are low not only in calories but in saturated fat as well.

TABLE 6:
FOOD FOR THOUGHT

Haddock	Turkey	Cabbage
Flounder	Mushrooms	Brussels sprouts
Sole	Asparagus	Carrots
Scallops	Lettuce	Cauliflower
Clams	Celery	Eggplant
Oysters	String beans	Onions
Chicken	Summer squash	

Fish is one of the best sources of protein that you can buy if you want to limit both cholesterol and calories. As I have previously noted, the oily fish should be avoided in favor of the many with a low fat content. Chicken and turkey are next for recommendation. Dark meat has more calories and more fat than white.

There is no question in the minds of most that the human body benefits by regular and controlled exercise. It certainly helps to keep the muscles in tone and the figure trim, it probably helps to prevent atherosclerosis, and it may even promote longevity. It is my impression, however, that the exercise fad, like most other fads in the past, is getting out of hand. For those who enjoy jogging and who can jog without jeopardizing their cardiopulmonary systems and joints, I endorse the effort. I am not as enthusiastic about the currently popular running events for which hundreds, even thousands, of people sign up to participate. Some are competent athletes who have conditioned themselves for such extreme energy expenditure, but most are at best no more than partially prepared for sustained exertion. I recently witnessed such a "mini-marathon" run. Participating were men and women, children and people old enough to know better. The distance was approximately six miles, and the expressions on the faces of most of the runners suggested that it was at least six miles too far. Competitive exercise where speed and endurance are factors is usually bad for health. It should be restricted to the young and the vigorous and those for whom machismo is a vital necessity. The rest of us should be more temperate.

Nonetheless, the problem of exercise eventually must be faced by everyone. Some people will exercise because they enjoy it. They are to be envied. Those who like and are good at competitive games—tennis, squash, handball, and the like—need no urging to use this means to keep fit. The drawback to this type of exercise is that it requires participation by others and that can mean the exercise is taken neither often nor regularly enough to be of value in maintaining health. An effective exercise program requires frequent and regular indulgence.

A number of regimens can be pursued alone and provide exercise that is steady and moderate. These include walking, golf (without a cart), swimming (leisurely), bowling, and bicycling. None requires great exertion or elaborate preparation. The calorie consumption is not great (about 1.5 calories per hour per pound of body weight), but no exercise is in itself a very effective means of weight reduction. Exercise provides rewards other than the burning of energy.

Far and away the best exercise for the average person is walking. It requires no special place or costume. Indeed, it does not even require a special time, because it can be combined with many routine duties such as going to and coming from work, shopping, or mowing the lawn. The lunch hour may be devoted to walking or the work itself may be incorporated into a walking regimen. Those who work in offices above ground level and who normally use the elevator have a built-in opportunity for a unique and wonderful type of exercise, climbing stairs, which can be exceedingly valuable if it is intelligently controlled. Walking on a level is also useful and beneficial. It is one of the finest exercises one can indulge in. Walking daily for from two to six miles at about four miles per hour with head up, shoulders back, chest high, and belly pulled in can do more for good health than most of the more exotic and elaborately planned programs.

A final note must be appended to this book: good health can rarely be achieved through taking drugs. As a physician, I should be the last to denigrate the use of those medications that correct or compensate for the deficiencies imposed by ill health. There are a number of drugs—antibiotics, vaccines, insulin, anesthetics, vitamins, and hormones—that are life saving. But it is a sad truth that almost half the drugs taken in our society provide no true benefits. Abuse is most blatant among a relatively small number: the sedatives (Valium particularly), laxatives, mind alterers (marijuana, LSD, heroin, cocaine, etc.), and, of course, alcohol and nicotine. Of these, alcohol, which has been viewed by the medical profession as a menace since the beginning of the century, is only now beginning to regain some respectability. Some recent evidence suggests that alcoholic beverages used in temperate amounts may help delay the progress of atherosclerosis. In the case of nicotine, there can be nothing but the sternest of condemnation. The fact that the cigarette habit almost certainly causes lung cancer is only the tip of the iceberg. It probably aids in and brings about a far greater number of deaths from cardiovascular causes than all the lung cancers for which it has been held responsible.

If this book needs a final admonition, it should read: refuse to eat the foods that are now purported to cause atherosclerosis, maintain a weight level compatible with the best longevity figures, have your total cholesterol/HDL ratio and your blood pressure checked periodically, use only drugs that promote health, exercise regularly and sensibly, drink moderately, and never smoke a cigarette.

19

Menus for a Healthy Heart

I have no illusions about my abilities as a chef. I have, however, in the preparation of this book drawn on the knowledge and advice of a number who are. Few of the recipes given here would be considered gourmet in character, although they may be used to enhance and supplement a gourmet meal. Nor have I attempted to make the following pages into a cookbook; there are already too many specialized cookbooks on the market. Rather, this chapter is intended to provide those who have a serious desire to preserve their health and prolong their lives with a number of menus and a few recipes that will help make an optimum diet easy and enjoyable.

There are two rules to keep in mind when designing such a menu. First, every food item in a diet must be evaluated on the basis of its saturated fat content and its number of calories. If you cannot obtain foods with a low score on both counts and you must, therefore, choose one or the other, it is preferable to select a high-caloric food rather than one that is fatty. Fat accumulated in the tissues can be reduced before it has done too much damage; atheromatous plaques, on the other hand, are probably permanent and by eating high-fat foods you may be contributing to the plaque that will close one of your coronary arteries, precipitating a situation that is permanent indeed.

The second rule is that the food chosen must be enjoyable. If it is not, the diet is scheduled for failure before it achieves anything of value. A bowl of bran flakes served with skimmed milk could be considered ideal fare on the basis of its fat and caloric values, but most people would prefer to suffer coronary occlusion than eat it on a daily basis. The fact is you can design an interesting and palatable diet if you are willing to discipline your taste buds a little. I know of no intelligent and unbiased person who would claim that the flavors of good fresh butter and imitation margarine are interchangeable. Until accustomed to the latter—that is, until the taste buds have become conditioned—there are few who would choose margarine in preference to butter on the basis of flavor alone. Given a valid reason and a few weeks trial, however, most unbiased people learn to accept the imitation without complaint although without, perhaps, great relish.

Salad Dressings

When we begin to think of menus, it is clear that one class of foods above all others must be used as infrequently as possible. These are fats of all kinds, especially saturated animal fats. This realization may fill the heart of the average cook with despair. How can one prepare a good sandwich without mayonnaise? How can one make all those wonderful sautéed vegetable and meat dishes without plenty of butter in the pan? How can one make pastry without lard, and what desserts are there without butter and eggs? A chef of the *nouvelle cuisine* would answer "Very good questions. It is a challenge, but it is not impossible." Let us begin with mayonnaise.

Because mayonnaise contains both egg yolks and oil, it is doubly damned. But an imitation mayonnaise *can* be made without egg yolks and with polyunsaturated oils. To be sure, the result is not real mayonnaise with its rich depth and subtle tang, but you may be surprised to find how good it is and how admirably it substitutes for the real thing.

I consider anyone who owns a blender and buys mayonnaise a willful spendthrift. Any child can make mayonnaise for less than half what store-bought costs. It takes a bit more skill and discernment to make a low-calorie, low-fat "mayonnaise" but it can be done.

A tablespoon of this low-fat imitation mayonnaise contains 75 calories of which only 15 calories are derived from fat. A very thick mixture is good to use on salads with wet ingredients or to make tartare sauce with capers or pickle relish, barbeque sauces with ketchup and Worcestershire sauce.

LOW-FAT IMITATION MAYONNAISE

1 c. oil (3 parts vegetable, 1 part heavy mineral)
2 egg whites
2 T. vinegar, lemon, or lime juice
1/2 t. salt (or 2 packages MBT)*
1/2 t. dry mustard
1/2 t. sugar
dash of pepper
1/2 t. curry powder (optional)
1/4 c. hot water (approximate)

All ingredients, with the exception of the water, should be at room temperature. Place one-quarter of the oil and all the remaining ingredients into a blender and mix at blend speed. While the blender is running, add the remainder of the oil, a few drops at a time at first and then in a thin stream. Stop the blender several times to scrape the mixture off the walls and around the blades with a rubber spatula. When the consistency is that of very soft butter, begin adding the hot water a little at a time. Alternate water and oil until the mixture attains the desired consistency. Place the mixture (still in the blender) in the refrigerator and allow to chill. When cold, note consistency. If too thick, remove from refrigerator, add more hot water, and blend until proper thickness is achieved. Yields 20 servings.

The idea of using mineral oil in preparation of salad dressings has been around for a long time. It had a period of popularity about fifty years ago when it was realized that

* MBT is a commercial broth concentrate powder. It comes in foil packets each containing 1 tablespoon. There are beef, chicken, and vegetable flavors, and each can be used as a substitute for salt.

mineral oil was not absorbed through the intestinal wall, which meant that those on a low-calorie diet could have their salad and eat it too. Unfortunately, most who tried it used it straight and in quantities that made the practice impractical. Many people with distasteful memories that stem from childhood experience with mineral oil as a laxative would not even taste a dressing if they knew it contained that oil. So the practice was dropped. It was not reinstated, perhaps because it was known that vitamins A and D are soluble in mineral oil. However, the quantity now recommended is insufficient to make this fact important. The use of mineral oil as a substitute for caloric oils merits another look. To the best of my knowledge, if used in the amounts suggested here even over long periods, it will cause no health problem.

Good mineral oil has no taste. I have made up a jar of mayonnaise using undiluted mineral oil only. Properly seasoned, this mixture is completely palatable and I was unable to distinguish it from a mayonnaise made entirely with vegetable oil. However if you wish to try mineral oil in your dressings, I suggest you start out by substituting only a quarter of the oil called for in the recipe with calorieless, nonatherogenic mineral oil. Below is the recipe for a light but piquant dressing.

One tablespoon of it contains about three grams of fat, almost all of which is polyunsaturated, and about thirty calories. These amounts may be compared with sixteen grams of fat, most of it saturated, and eighty-six calories per tablespoon of a number of commercial salad dressings. This dressing takes only a few moments to make, it is cheaper than its commercial competitors, and it is quite palatable. Its character is readily varied by adding more mustard, chopped onion, celery seed or any other ingredient that may strike your fancy. It does tend to thicken when kept in the refrigerator more than two or three days, but adding a little water and blending for a few seconds will restore its texture.

You can further decrease the fat and calories in this dressing by using one tablespoon of mineral with three of vegetable oil. Each one-tablespoon serving of this dressing contains about a fifth of a teaspoon of mineral oil. This amount, even if taken daily, should not cause symptoms in anyone.

SALAD DRESSING

1 c. water
1/4 c. oil (preferably sunflower, corn may be used)
4 T. vinegar
2 T. powdered pectin
1 t. prepared mustard (hot)
1 t. salt
1 t. sugar
1 t. garlic powder (optional)
dash black pepper

Place all ingredients in a blender and combine at high speed. Yields approximately one cup of creamy liquid.

Some cooks increase the body of their mayonnaise by adding powdered gelatin. The result is pretty much what you would expect it to be, a quivering bowl of something that acts and tastes more like Jell-O than salad dressing.

Another thickened dressing relies on cornstarch to supply body. This dressing contains no eggs, but it must be cooked. The original was called "boiled dressing." It used no oil and only a few egg yolks. I have stretched this concept a bit further to exclude eggs entirely. It is surprisingly palatable. The fat content is negligible; the calories for the whole, 180, about 20 per one-tablespoon serving. Do not expect a rich mayonnaise flavor, but this dressing is worthy if only for variation.

BOILED SALAD DRESSING

1 1/2 c. nonfat dry milk
2 T. cornstarch
1/4 c. vinegar
2 t. prepared mustard
1 t. salt

In a double boiler, stir the milk into the cornstarch a little at a time to make a paste and then a liquid. Stir constantly while cooking the mixture over slow heat until it is thick and clear. Mix the vinegar, mustard, and salt in a bowl and add to milk and cornstarch. When it is hot but before it boils, pour into a jar and refrigerate. Yields approximately one pint.

A vinaigrette dressing can be concocted if you want to avoid oil entirely.

VINAIGRETTE DRESSING

1/2 c. vinegar (lemon or lime juice may be substituted)
1/4 c. water
2 T. sugar (or to taste)
2 T. sweet pickle juice
1 t. salt
garlic powder to taste
pepper to taste

Shake well in a bottle with a stopper.

A creamy variation of the vinaigrette, called tangy cream dressing, contains more calories (about 100 total); but they are derived from protein and carbohydrate, and the fat content is negligible.

TANGY CREAM DRESSING

1/4 c. yogurt, low fat
2 T. vinegar
2 T. prepared mustard (hot)
1 T. sugar
2 T. dill weed, dried
salt and pepper to taste

Combine all ingredients and blend.

Frying and Substitute Methods

We now come to the problem of frying, probably the oldest, certainly the simplest, cooking technique. It would be impossible to eradicate it no matter how bad its press. People will always fry, but intelligent people will abandon deep-frying forever. If the cholesterol-conscious dieter were to make but one resolution, the most valuable one he could choose would be never to eat anything that is deep-fried. Treatment of the most delectable and innocent foods in this manner more than doubles their caloric count and makes their fat content prohibitive. No, deep-frying should be forbidden, completely and forever. There are techniques that can be substituted. They will not produce exactly the same results but neither will they produce atherosclerosis, obesity, and peptic ulcer.

A number of products on the market enable us to "fry" food without adding fat yet avoiding having it stick to the pan. These "no-stick" products, which are marketed under a variety of names and usually packaged in spray cans, are principally lecithin complexes. Press the button on the top of the can and a blast of this material spreads itself over the inside of the pan, the object to be fried, and if one is not very careful, over various objects in range. It also blows the breading off the food that is being treated and after a couple of usages it often forms a sticky gum over the aperture that permanently blocks the passage of the can's contents. Despite these minor faults, these products are effective and should be used.

Other tactics should be tried. The appearance and flavor of many fried foods have been traditionally enhanced by breading. But breading need not necessarily lead to deep-frying. It can be used to create delicious low-fat dishes just as easily, if done properly. Choose from a variety of crumbs made from various kinds of breads, crackers, or cornflakes. If bread is used, the crumbs should be made fresh in the blender. Sourdough bread or English muffins make a coarse breading that is especially good. Breading two portions of fish or meat requires an egg white and a slice of bread, adding about 100 calories to the meal.

First, dry the item to be breaded. Dust lightly with flour either by rolling in a plate of flour or shaking in a paper bag. Next, dip in a liquid made of egg white beaten lightly with two tablespoons of water. Finally, roll in crumbs.

The most important maneuver in the breading process is the drying interval. Lay the breaded pieces on a rack for thirty minutes or longer before cooking. Failure to do so may result in loss of most of the coating in the pan.

To prevent sticking and promote browning, moisten the bottom of a cake or cookie tin with a few drops of vegetable oil spread in a thin coating with fingertips or a paper towel. Lay the breaded, dried pieces in the pan and drizzle two or three drops of oil on each side of each piece. This is done most conveniently by using a plastic bottle the tin cap of which has been perforated with an ice pick. Mineral oil can be used satisfactorily although it has a tendency to smoke. Cook in a 450-degree oven until nicely browned.

The results of this technique approach those of deep-frying more closely than any other I know. The oven must be very hot when the food is put in, and the cooking time must not be prolonged beyond that necessary for optimum flavor. If this method is used, the added fat is minimal and the caloric increase over that of the unadorned main ingredients is barely appreciable.

Desserts

Most desserts are rich in fats and heavy in calories and many are both. Because there is no sane substitute for such desserts they must be deleted from the diet of anyone striving to avoid atherosclerosis and obesity. Pies and cakes of all types and other pastries made with butter or lard are out of the question. Desserts made with egg yolks, such as puddings, custards, and flans, are also forbidden. Chocolate is rich in saturated fats; nuts are high in calories. Ice cream made with cream is obviously taboo. Most commercial ice creams contain little real cream, but they may be made with substitutes that are worse, or they may contain carbohydrate thickeners that are laden with calories. It is probably best to avoid all ice cream. Most sherbets contain so much sugar that they should not be eaten without due consideration of their caloric content. In this category, only the fruit ices are reasonably safe. You may well ask what is left. The answer is very little.

If you examine the many books on diet cookery available today, you may be surprised to find that little space is devoted to desserts. Most books suggest fresh fruit and then wash their hands of the matter. Perhaps that is the best policy. Fresh fruit of one kind or another is almost always available and most make acceptable desserts, particularly melons, which have no fat content and are usually low in calories. A quarter of a large cantaloupe contains only about thirty-five calories. A squeeze of lime juice will brighten the flavor of many of these fruits. Topping fresh fruit with unsweetened low-fat yogurt (with perhaps some vanilla extract stirred in) will add a sense of richness to a low-calorie dessert.

Because cheeses contain large amounts of fat and are high in casein, only such low-fat cheeses as Parmesan and provolone can be recommended in cooking and in small quantities at that. For the same reason, they should not be eaten indiscriminately in sandwiches and the like. A small piece of cheese (1½ cubic inches) such as Camembert or Roquefort may be enjoyed with an apple for dessert. Some cheeses are gourmet delights; it would be a great pity to abandon them entirely, so here I will make an exception, although I admit it is a personal indulgence. Some people can be induced to substitute yogurt for cheese; others would prefer to go without dessert. One of the most delightful ways to end a good meal is with an excellent piece of cheese, a crust of fresh French bread, a few seedless grapes, and a glass of dessert wine such as Asti spumanti. This fare is too regal for gross consumption and so the fats and calories are kept at a minimum. And I insist on thinking, without much scientific reason, that the alcohol of the wine will counteract the fat of the cheese.

Recently, a number of brands of what are generally called nondairy creamers have come on the market. They look like very heavy cream and, if one is not too discerning, taste quite like it. This product was originally meant to be stirred into coffee; but its popularity has broadened to use in cooking, especially in sauces, soups, and gravies. It does give a creamy consistency and a rich flavor. Furthermore, it is reasonably cheap and will stay fresh in the refrigerator for weeks. Those that I have examined claim to contain no dairy products. The ones whose formulas I have been able to obtain are made predominantly of coconut oil and casein and are probably more damaging to your aorta than pure rich cream would be. I would not use any of these substances unless the formula is printed on the container to assure that the contents have less saturated fat than the dairy product for which they are meant to substitute.

Meal Planning

A number of diet books are made up entirely of specific menus for each meal of the day, each day of the week, and each week of the year. They must be written for people completely without will, without taste, and I suspect without individuality. We are not an ant colony. In the following pages I make some suggestions concerning the diet you should be eating. I provide routine menus only to illustrate the manner in which you may make your own. The suggestions are for those who have achieved the weight they wish to maintain. If you want to lose weight, consult the preceding chapters to learn how to design a reducing diet.

I assume that you have established your optimum weight and wish to maintain it on a diet that will prevent the development or progress of atherosclerosis. This means that not more than 25 percent of your daily calories may come from fats, and these fats shall be largely polyunsaturated. If you must be indiscreet it is better to take your excess calories from proteins and carbohydrates. Be aware, though, that it is impossible to eat too much beef, pork, or lamb protein without eating much animal fat, because the muscle and fat cells are so intimately related.

Suppose that you have calculated the number of calories that you should consume in order to maintain your weight (see Chapters 14 and 15) and you have made the proper additions for a controlled exercise program. If the number is 2,000, not more than 500 of these calories may come from fats. If you are a male of 5′11″ with medium frame, you should weigh about 146 pounds. With ordinary exercise you will require around 2,500 calories daily to maintain this weight. If you are a female of 5′8″ you should weigh about 128 pounds, and you will require around 2,000 calories. The following suggestions are calculated on a maintenance caloric intake of 2,000 calories. You should make corrections to satisfy your specific needs.

Suppose you eat three meals a day. If you insist on morning or afternoon snacks then you must subtract these caloric indiscretions from your regular meal allowance. To establish a framework for your calculations, you might divide your daily caloric budget into 300 calories for breakfast, 700 for lunch and

1,000 for dinner. In order to make calculations easy to keep track of, round off figures. For example, an ordinary bowl of dry cereal with sugar and skimmed milk varies from 120 to 175 calories. It is permissible to round off the figure to 150 so that you need not remember the exact number of calories in each cereal type.

Breakfast

Breakfast is important more in terms of what you may not do than what you may. Many people are bored by the rather monotonous and uninteresting fare of an approved breakfast and prefer to skip this part of the daily ritual and take a cup of coffee on the run or at their desk. I can find no health reason to disagree with these people. Most of us have been brought up on the dictum that a growing child and a working man must start the day with a hot and nourishing meal. I doubt that. Some of nature's strongest and hardiest creatures (lions, for example) rarely eat more often than once a day, and sometimes only once in two or three days. In most of us, our physiology is geared to span many hours without ingesting food. The headaches that occur on an empty stomach are largely psychological in origin and disappear when the sufferer understands its mechanism. Occasionally (and not nearly as often as we are told), the blood sugar will fall below a critical level, inducing fatigue. When this occurs, a quick snack of highly refined sugar (candy or a sweet drink) will usually restore the afflicted to normal.

At breakfast time there are four nevers: eggs, bacon, ham, and sausage. If you must indulge yourself at this time of day, pile in a platter of buckwheat pancakes with maple syrup (watch the butter) but no eggs, bacon, ham, or sausage. They are gone forever, except perhaps on Christmas and your birthday. If you insist on breakfast, you may have some juice—tomato or vegetable—or a piece of fruit—half a grapefruit or quarter of melon—for around 50 calories. Most orange juice, fresh or frozen, comes a bit higher, particularly if it is sweetened. An artificial sweetener goes well on grapefruit. If you like toast, you may have two thin slices with imitation margarine and a tablespoon of marmalade or jam. The kind of bread (as long as it is thinly sliced at about 50 calories each) does not matter as much as our bakers would like us to think—choose the type that tastes best. This combination with all the black coffee or tea you feel like drinking comes to around 300 calories. There is little excuse to use sugar in coffee. Each teaspoon adds 20 calories to your meal and cavities to your teeth. With a little self-discipline you will find sweetened coffee anathema. If black coffee is too strong, add a little nonfat milk.

Many people insist on a dry cereal for breakfast. They have a valid reason although, I insist, an unimaginative sense of taste. An accumulating body of evidence suggests that we are better off with a certain percentage of fiber food in our diets. Highly refined sugars have been linked with atherosclerosis and fiber foods do substitute for these calories. Bulk also enhances elimination, whereas a high protein diet with little fiber invites stagnation. Bowel cancer is more common in societies on high-protein, low-roughage diets. Nonetheless, coarse-fiber foods must be used with caution, particularly by those with a penchant for peptic ulcer.

Lunch

We cannot begin to review even a fair sample of the vast array of possibilities that are available for lunch. I believe the meal should be light, unless you prefer your main meal at midday and a *light* supper in the evening. In Hispanic countries the large meal is usually taken at about two in the afternoon followed by a siesta during the hottest part of the day. Work is resumed in mid-afternoon and continues into the evening. The evening meal is therefore late, often not before ten o'clock. The diner usually retires soon after his supper. A nap of about an hour on a full stomach is a part of nature's ritual—most animals take one if allowed—but a busy stomach is not conducive to a good night's rest. An hour or two of activity is recommended before attempting serious repose.

Probably the two most common lunches in this country are soup and a sandwich or a salad and sandwich. In terms of their calorie content, soups fall into three categories: the creamed soups with a calorie count of around 200 per bowl; broths with approximately 100 calories; and bouillons that contain from 10 to 30 calories. A fourth type, those made with beans and meats, are too high in calories (about 300) but not in fat. Most vegetable soups, including uncreamed tomato and pea, contain around 100 calories per bowl. Clear chicken broth usually has a little more than 100. Good beef broth, however, is very high in fat and should be avoided. The bouillons prepared from powdered concentrates are good to have around for a diet; a cup contains about 10 calories and offers a degree of solace to the deprived palate.

Almost anything in the kitchen can be used to fill a sandwich. Time-honored favorites include white meat of chicken, lean beef, or the so-called lunch meats—boiled ham, salami, bologna, and other sausages. These last are usually compounded of fatty meat trimmings which puts them off-limits. Liver sausage (Braunschweiger) is an exception. It is high in calories, but its fat content is within acceptable limits. Baked and fried ham are forbidden, but when boiled and sliced very thin it is acceptable if all the apparent fat is carefully dissected away. It isn't when the sandwich is prepared at the average lunch counter. Thin slices of cold roast beef may be treated in the same manner. A chicken sandwich is probably the best bet for steady consumption. For the determined dieter, there is always the lettuce and tomato sandwich with a calorie count of around 200.

All sandwiches should be made on thinly sliced bread and spread with imitation margarine, home-made diet mayonnaise, or mustard. All the above suggestions can be made in a palatable form with fewer than 300 calories and about a 20 percent fat content.

Salads vary almost as much as sandwiches. Because most salads are prepared largely with lettuce, chopped cabbage (cole slaw), or other raw vegetables, the caloric total of the main constituent is usually above suspicion; it is the dressing that counts. Forego the commercial preparations and try some of the salad dressings and mayonnaise described earlier in this chapter.

All of these lunch suggestions, combinations of soup and sandwich or salad and sandwich, when prepared according to the rules, will add up to fewer than 700 calories, even when a glass of skimmed milk is added. Indeed, if you choose a 200 calorie soup and a 300 calorie sandwich, you can also include a salad if you feel hungry. The person on an intelligent diet need not leave the lunch table craving food. In none of the suggested combinations does the fat percentage rise above acceptable limits.

Dinner

What follows are menus for two ordinary dinners to illustrate the practical aspects of regular meal planning with low-fat and low-calorie foods. Each dinner consists of a meat, two vegetables, and a modest dessert. Because the meals are simple the portions are generous, about seven ounces of meat and three and a half ounces of each vegetable. Both meals may be accompanied by an eight-ounce glass of skimmed milk and contain fewer than 1,000 calories of which less than 25 percent is derived from fat.

DINNER A

Chicken with béchamel, braised mushrooms, broccoli in tangy cream sauce, fruit sherbet, and black coffee.

Chicken. Use two *suprêmes* (skinless and boneless half-breasts) or two thighs per serving. A *suprême* should always be cooked as follows. Use a flameproof, ovenproof pot with a lid. Preheat the oven to 375 degrees. While the pan is heating on top of the stove, cut a piece of waxed paper the size of the lid and grease one surface with oil or imitation margarine. Put just enough polyunsaturated oil in the pan to cover the bottom. When the pan is very hot, lay in the *suprêmes* and watch for color to appear, about a minute. Do not allow them to brown. Turn and cook on the other side for no longer than a minute. Drop the circle of waxed paper, oiled side down, onto the *suprêmes* and press it down firmly into place; put the lid on and put the pot in the preheated oven for exactly six minutes. The center of the *suprême* should have just the faintest blush of pink; overcooking makes it tough. If you are using thighs, bread and oven-bake them as described on page 163. In either case serve with the following sauce.

This simple béchamel is made in a double boiler. Use four tablespoons of unsaturated vegetable oil and add two tablespoons of flour. Stir to a heavy paste. Slowly add half a cup of skimmed milk, stirring constantly to a creamy consistency. Add salt and pepper to taste and a quarter cup of vermouth, either dry or sweet. Stir in one half packet of Butter Buds. Add the liquid from the pan the *suprêmes* were cooked in. If the sauce is too thick, thin it with vermouth; if it is too thin, it can be thickened with a little cornstarch to which a tablespoon of water has been added.

The flavor of this sauce can be varied with almost anything that comes to mind: green pepper corns, lemon juice, lobster bits, curry powder, chopped black olives, pimientos. It has a sunny and obliging temperament and accepts almost any treatment without protest.

Mushrooms. Select the largest and freshest on the market. Do not buy small, broken, or withered ones. Separate the caps from the stems by breaking with your fingers. It is a simple procedure to peel the caps. Simply lift the underedge with your fingers and pull toward the center. The stems and peelings can be boiled up together for sauces and soups.

Heat the heaviest pan in your kitchen on top of the stove until it is very hot. Use just enough vegetable oil to cover the bottom. Throw in the caps and cook rapidly, shaking the pan and stirring constantly. The entire procedure should not take more than a minute and a half. Remove to a heated bowl and season to taste with salt (or bouillon powder), black pepper, powdered garlic (if desired) and a half packet of Butter Buds. These seasonings do not stand up well under intense heat.

Broccoli. All green vegetables should be blanched in ten times their volume of furiously boiling water the moment they are brought from the market or garden. This inactivates the enzymes and ensures that the vegetables will taste as though they had just been picked even if you cook them several days later. Even sweet corn should be treated in this manner.

To cook preblanched broccoli, split the stems and boil in just enough salted water to cover for about ten minutes. The age of the plant determines the time of the cooking. Test for a crisp yet tender consistency. Drain and serve either hot or cold with tangy cream dressing (page 162).

The entire meal, with a fruit sherbet dessert, adds up to just about 1,000 calories of which less than 25 percent is derived from fat.

DINNER B

Flounder or haddock, asparagus, gingered carrots, melon.

Fish. The fish filets may be fresh or frozen. They should be as thin as they can be cut. Thick slices must be cooked longer and cooking makes fish tough. Dry each piece and dust it with flour. Dip in egg white mixture and bread as described on page 163. Lightly oil the breaded and dried pieces and place in a very heavy, very hot frying pan the bottom of which has been coated with a nonstick spray or the thinnest possible layer of oil. Cook on the top of the stove a matter of seconds on each side until the fish becomes nicely browned. Serve with a tartare sauce made with three-quarters of a cup of diet mayonnaise (page 159) to which a teaspoon of any or all of the following is added: chopped onion, pickle relish, capers, olives, chopped parsley. Or, the fish may be accompanied by a relish such as the following: two cups of finely chopped cabbage and two medium-size green peppers mixed with one teaspoon of celery seed, a quarter of a teaspoon of mustard seed, two tablespoons of brown sugar, half a teaspoon of salt and a quarter of a teaspoon of vinegar. Allow the mixture to stand at room temperature a few hours before serving.

Asparagus. Take advantage of the jumbo stalks of California asparagus that are on the market for two or three weeks during the spring. Boil in enough water to cover until just tender when tested with a sharp fork. Overcooking changes the taste and makes the asparagus soft. Serve with imitation margarine and optional lemon juice.

Gingered carrots. Cover the bottom of a heavy pan with oil. Heat on top of the stove and add about three-quarters of a cup of sliced carrots per serving. Add one tablespoon of sugar, a splash of sweet vermouth, and two tablespoons of chopped candied ginger. Cook slowly for about half an hour or until the carrots are tender. Just before serving add a tablespoon of imitation margarine.

This meal may be finished off with a generous portion of melon and still have a margin of calories that should allow an accompanying glass of wine or, if you prefer, a cocktail before.

The details of these two dinners were given to illustrate how easy it is to design menus with the proper amounts of interesting and palatable food you should be eating. Armed with the knowledge of what you want to weigh and the number of calories it requires to maintain that weight, with a good kitchen scale and a manual of tables of fat content and calories, and with a bit of motivation and willingness to try the new low-fat preparations, anyone can eat well and healthfully. If a longer and healthier life is your objective, the effort is more than worthwhile.

Index